The
Thinking Person's
Guide
to Diabetes

The Thinking Person's Guide to Diabetes

THE DRAZNIN PLAN

Boris Draznin, MD, PhD

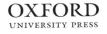

OXFORD
UNIVERSITY PRESS

2003

OXFORD

UNIVERSITY PRESS

Oxford   New York
Auckland   Bangkok   Buenos Aires   Cape Town   Chennai
Dar es Salaam   Delhi   Hong Kong   Istanbul   Karachi   Kolkata
Kuala Lumpur   Madrid   Melbourne   Mexico City   Mumbai
Nairobi   São Paulo   Shanghai   Taipei   Tokyo   Toronto

Published by Oxford University Press, Inc.
198 Madison Avenue, New York, New York, 10016
http://www.oup-usa.org

Oxford is a registered trademark of Oxford University Press

Library of Congress Cataloging-in-Publication Data
Draznin, Boris.
The thinking person's guide to diabetes :
the Draznin plan /
by Boris Draznin.
p. cm.   Includes index.
ISBN 0-19-516740-6
1. Non-insulin-dependent diabetes—Popular works.
2. Weight loss—Popular works.
I. Title.
RC662.18.D73 2003   616.4'62—dc21   2003041934

While the advice and information in this book are believed to be true and accurate at the date of going to press, neither the author nor the publisher can accept any responsibility or liability for any errors or omissions that may be made. In particular, note that drug dosage schedules are constantly being revised and new side effects recognized. The publisher and the author make no representation, express or implied, that the drug dosages in this book are correct. For these reasons, readers are strongly urged to consult their physicians and the drug company's printed instructions before taking any drugs.

To protect confidentiality, all patient names in this book are fictional, and certain details of their stories may have been changed. In addition, case descriptions may be composites of several cases.

This book is meant solely for informational purposes. It is not intended that any of the ideas, procedures, or suggestions mentioned here be regarded as substitutes for expert medical services where they are required.

2 4 6 8 9 7 5 3 1

Printed in the United States of America
on acid-free paper

Preface

Not a week passes by without a story about an epidemic of obesity and Type 2 diabetes in the United States. These stories appear regularly either in one of the major national news publications or by being broadcast by one of the television networks. This epidemic is not limited to the U.S. borders; Canada, England, and other industrialized nations are experiencing these same intractable health problems.

This epidemic is real. It is frightening. It has colossal implications for the health of our population and for the health-care system in general. Obesity and Type 2 diabetes are silent killers responsible for the shortened life expectancy of many patients. One of the most important complications of Type 2 diabetes is acceleration and progression of cardiovascular disease, leading to heart attack and stroke. Needless to say, these complications significantly and adversely affect both the life span and quality of life.

At the same time, clinical trials have convincingly demonstrated that Type 2 diabetes can be prevented. Modifications in eating and activity patterns effectively prevented diabetes in almost 60% of "prediabetic" patients. We have also learned that weight reduction helps control blood pressure and cholesterol problems. The old adage about "an ounce of prevention" goes far beyond its true wisdom when it is applied to weight problems and diabetes. Prevention of Type 2 diabetes literally saves lives.

Understanding the problem does not necessarily mean that a solution is at hand. Losing weight and maintaining this new "reduced" appearance is far from being a trivial task. The sheer number of books offering "a simple and quick" weight-loss recipe tells me (and, it is hoped, you) that the problem is much more complex than these books imply. Otherwise, we would have solved this problem long ago. The truth is—there is no single recipe. Weight maintenance requires a long-term commitment to a different (therapeutic) lifestyle.

Diabetes and obesity are two chronic conditions that cannot be cured or even controlled without the patient's involvement. The Draznin Plan offers help to those who are ready and willing to get involved. My plan is based upon three principles: scientific facts, an individualized approach, and unwavering commitment to lifestyle changes. The lifestyle changes presented in my book will help you attain your goals—to improve or prevent Type 2 diabetes and maintain a healthy weight. However, only the combined efforts of the Draznin Plan and your personal commitment to my recommendations will bear the desired fruit.

Denver, Colorado   B. D.

Contents

Chapter 9
TREATMENT OF OBESITY, 95

Chapter 10
THE DRAZNIN CALORIE: A BETTER WAY TO DIET, 113

Chapter 11
PRACTICAL ADVICE, 123

Chapter 12
CASE STUDIES AND A TREATMENT PLAN FOR
MR. K, 147

Chapter 13
RECOMMENDATIONS BASED ON TEN DRAZNIN
RULES OF LIFE, 167

Chapter 14
FREQUENTLY ASKED QUESTIONS, 173

INDEX, 185

The
Thinking Person's
Guide
to Diabetes

A Letter
to
My Reader

Dear Reader,

When you took my book from the shelf in your favorite bookstore or library, you may have wondered what is so special about my program. In what way is Dr. Draznin's approach better than dozens of others staring at you from the same bookshelf? What is the secret of the Draznin Plan that allows his patients to defeat their obesity and Type 2 diabetes?[1]

Not only do I encourage you to ask these questions, but also I hope you find the answers in my book convincing and reassuring. I believe firmly that the more people understand about their weight problems and dia-

1. Type 2 diabetes is the most common form of diabetes, frequently associated with excess weight and insulin resistance (inadequate action of insulin). See Chapter 6 for more detail.

betes, the greater their participation will be, and the greater their chances for success.

In many cases, weight maintenance and prevention of Type 2 diabetes are, at least in part, in the hands of patients themselves, and my role is simply to guide them through the obstacle course of energy intake and energy expenditure.

Having treated thousands of patients with diabetes and obesity for over three decades of academic medical practice, I have developed a unique program: the Draznin Plan. It is built on a solid scientific foundation, is easy to understand and follow, and has proven successful by patients who made a true commitment to their lifestyle changes.

The Draznin Plan is based on three principles, "a three-legged stool," if you will. The first is the science of clinical medicine, nowadays known as "evidence-based medicine." The cardinal feature of contemporary Western medicine is its reliance on controlled clinical studies to identify which treatments work and which ones do not. Anecdotal success stories, individual experiences with exotic therapies, and the popularity of nontraditional practitioners cannot substitute for the rigor of clinical research with appropriate control groups and scientific statistical analysis. Only proven therapies should be accepted as standards of care.

The field of weight maintenance is not an exception. Numerous clinical studies have repeatedly shown that any person on a low-calorie diet is going to lose weight. Interestingly, however, exercise without an accompanying diet failed to produce significant weight loss. Thus, telling patients that they can lose weight simply by increasing their energy expenditure would be misleading. In contrast, other studies have convincingly demonstrated that, after an initial weight loss, only those individuals who have incorporated exercise into their lifestyles have been able to maintain their reduced weight. The others regained their pounds.

These studies are telling us that neither a low-calorie diet without exercise nor exercise without a low-calorie diet is adequate for long-term success in weight maintenance. This is why a combination of the Draznin Mile and the Draznin Calorie work together.

The second principle of my approach lies in its individualized design. We are all distinct human beings, with our very own personalized abilities to follow directions, maintain a program, and engage in physical activities. Each of us has our own taste and food preferences, work schedule, lifestyle, and recreational interests. Going to a doctor's office, we expect an individualized approach to our medical problems. I, for example, expect my physician to identify my problems specifically and treat them accordingly.

Otherwise, I could just walk into a pharmacy and buy over-the-counter medications. Occasionally, we all do just that, but, in most cases, I want my doctor to do an examination, to find out why I cough, and to prescribe medications that are right for me. No two problems are identical, even though many are alike. No two patients are the same, even though they may have similar problems or symptoms.

We should not settle for anything less in the treatment of obesity and diabetes. This individualized approach is the second leg of this "three-legged stool."

The last and, unfortunately, the weakest leg of this tripod is your own commitment to lifestyle changes, my dear reader. That is where most programs fail. That is why, as the May 2002 issue of *Consumer Reports* stated, less than 25% of all dieters were able to keep their weight down for a year, regardless of the diet they had used.

You, my reader, should be ready to embark on a journey along a very different lifestyle, and I (my book, to be precise) will be your skipper, helping you maintain your new course. I offer to your attention the most practical guide and the most realistic approach to your problems with weight maintenance. Over a hundred of my patients have used my plan and over 80% of them achieved their goals.

This is not a prescription for exercise. I am well aware that you are tired of being urged to exercise. I understand that you, my reader, cannot become an athlete or a spokesperson in a commercial for an exercise machine.

Nor does my approach consist of a set of recipes. The last thing you need is more recipes. Your bookshelf is already sagging under the weight of cookbooks and recipe books. You are a normal, living being, a reasonably active person, who is not sweating in a gym or pedaling miles of bike trails. You work, you take care of your home and your family, and you are mildly-to-moderately overweight. You wish to lose about 10 pounds, and to drop one or two clothing sizes. You wish to stay healthy.

The Draznin Plan will be an eye-opener for you. This is exactly what you need, to guide you to your goals. I have developed a practical and commonsense concept that will help you modify your lifestyle, your pattern of activity, and your eating habits in order to attain your goals.

All of us, or better said, almost all with rare exceptions, love a hearty and tasty meal. Delicious and savory food is both pleasure and fun. Eating should be a joy. Eating out is frequently an event. Good breakfast defines our day. A lovely picnic with friends is a lively entertainment. An elegant dinner is a wonderful night-cap. A diet, regardless of its composition, is an antonym of good living. A diet is a drag, a constant fight with guilt and frustration, a perpetual struggle. Why, then, do I recommend it to you? There is only one reason to do so—to improve your health and, possibly, longevity. This is why only when you come to this very conclusion will you be successful in maintaining your diet, provided the diet offers variety, taste, and satiety. The Draznin Plan has it all.

My program will empower you to be in charge of your weight—and your diabetes, if you have it. It relies on simplicity, long-term goals, patience, and adjustments. Realistic expectations will become your guiding principles. I am confident that my down-to-earth concept will help you change your lifestyle forever.

Finally, here comes the most important question you might ask: "Why should I buy your book, Dr. Draznin?"

Excellent question. And here is my four-point answer: First, and most important, my book offers practical commonsense advice that will allow you to adopt the Draznin Plan into your daily living so as to achieve and maintain weight loss as well as to treat and prevent diabetes.

Second, my book describes numerous real-life illustrative cases that will aid you in your quest for meaningful lifestyle changes.

Third, my book provides a scientific background, for those who wish to explore it, describing how body weight is regulated and how we can therapeutically impact these regulatory mechanisms.

Finally, this book is written by a world-renowned authority on diabetes and metabolic disorders, a Professor of Medicine at a major university, one of the leading diabetologists in the United States, and an author of many scientific articles, book chapters, and monographs in this field.

Sincerely,

Boris Draznin, MD, PhD
Professor of Medicine
University of Colorado Health Sciences Center
Director of Research
Denver Veterans Affairs Medical Center

An
Introductory
Case

He who would eat the kernel must crack the nut.

"I'm about fifty pounds overweight, I have high blood pressure, and my doctor told me I have a great deal of risk in developing diabetes," announced Mr. Jeffrey K., from his chair in my office. Jeff was 6 feet tall, and weighed just over 230 pounds. His shoulders slouched forward as he bent over his bulging belly. His left ankle rested over his right knee; this was because he could no longer cross his legs owing to a protruding stomach. "In short," he continued, after taking a deep breath, "I've been welcomed to the club. This is the first time in my life I have to actively resist joining a club—a club of obese diabetics. Can you help me?"

Jeff was wrong. He wasn't about to join this "exclusive" club. He had already joined it; a club of 28 million Americans who are overweight, and 16 million Americans who have diabetes. His fasting blood-sugar level was 136 mg/dl (milligrams per deciliter), a full 26 points higher than the upper limit of the normal range, in the diagnostic criteria for diabetes.[1]

Jeffrey K. was a forty-seven-year-old successful lawyer, a "guru" in international business law, with strong entrepreneurial skills. He spoke fluent French and some German, and spent about 60% of his time in Europe and Africa, attending to business deals.

Hotel breakfast buffets, business lunches, and dinners had been his main diet for a number of years. Even back at home, he loved to take his family out to eat. He enjoyed ethnic foods and cold draft beer.

The fact that he was gaining weight steadily was fairly obvious to him, but Jeff didn't like to think about it. A couple of times, he had thought he should eat a bit less, but he loved his food so much that the very idea of dieting was simply foreign to him.

Jeff had never been very athletic, but in his college days he had loved to play touch-football and softball. He even thought he was quite good at these sports. He hadn't done anything in the way of exercise, however, since his days at law school.

He had known that many of the hotels where he stayed during his travels had health clubs, but he had never ventured out to any of them. He didn't feel like getting up early in the morning, and he was too tired, after a long working day, to exercise in the afternoon.

---

1. Normal fasting blood sugar levels range between 70 and 110 mg/ dl. Fasting blood sugar levels greater than 126 mg/dl define diabetes. Levels between 110 and 126 mg/dl are designated as "impaired fasting glucose."

"Mr. K.," I replied, politely, but firmly, "you do have diabetes. As you just pointed out, you also have obesity, the second largest preventable cause of premature death in this country. Only smoking causes more preventable deaths. There is a substantial probability that you can reverse your diabetes if you lose weight and return to a more active lifestyle. Not a guarantee, but you have a great chance for success.

"I have been doing research in diabetes, and treating patients with diabetes and weight problems, for more than thirty years," I continued. "These years of experience have allowed me to create and refine my own program, and it has helped many patients like yourself change their lifestyles, lose weight, and prevent the development of diabetes.

"You will have to eat less than you do now," I stressed, "and you will have to be much more active than you are now. I will teach you to exercise, so that you will be able to walk up to three Draznin Miles a day, and to eat up to eighteen Draznin Calories a day. I will also teach you where and what to eat when you dine out, how not to be hungry, and how to make physical activity a part of your life.

"The only way I can be of help to you, however, is if you and I reach a contract, which will require that you become an active participant in our efforts to restore your health. It won't be easy, and it won't be quick. You and I will have to introduce a lot of changes into your lifestyle, your attitude, and your commitment to health. I will guide you, but you will have to do the climbing to achieve our goal. I'll shed the light, but you'll have to walk the path. There are plenty of difficulties and frustrations along the way. You won't succeed unless you are totally dedicated to this goal. I cannot promise a cure, but, with your effort and commitment, we will certainly make significant improvement in your health and, consequently, longevity.

"Our success is in your hands," I concluded.

Jeff listened attentively, trying to guess what kind of changes he would have to implement, how much frustration he would have to endure, how much commitment he would have to make, and how much trust he would have to put in me and my program.

"You are a successful businessman, Mr. K.," I continued, reading his thoughts in his expression. "The word 'failure' is not in your vocabulary. And the reason you don't fail is very simple: It is because of your commitment to your business, your adherence to your plans, your perseverance in pursuing your goals and objectives, your ability to take one step at a time, making adjustments as you move along, and your vision of the future. You and I both know that you have to possess these exceptional qualities to navigate in the business world. What we must do is apply the same qualities to your lifestyle, exactly as you have applied them to your business.

"I am going to offer you a set of rules. I don't know whether you will live longer if you follow the Draznin rules, but I am certain that you'll increase your chances for longevity and undoubtedly enhance the quality of your life."

For several moments we sat in silence, looking straight into each other's eyes.

"You have three options," I said, with a smile, attempting to make it easier for Jeff. "You can leave this office right now and continue with your current lifestyle. You can spend an hour with me, hear my advice, and do with it whatever you wish. Take it or leave it, so to speak.

Or, finally, you can decide to make a commitment to your own health, and work with me to improve it."

Jeff pondered the options I offered him. We'll return to his reply later in the book. Meanwhile, let me tell you a little bit about myself and acquaint you with the Draznin rules of life.

I am a Professor of Medicine, Endocrinology, Diabetes, and Metabolism at the University of Colorado Health Sciences Center. My interest in diabetes may have been aroused by my own family history. My grandfather, my mother, and a maternal uncle had Type 2 diabetes. For over thirty years, from the day I finished medical school, I have been doing clinical and basic research in the field of diabetes, studying how insulin works and how to achieve the best control of this chronic disease. I have also been trying to find the best dietary regimen for my patients. In the process, I have developed an approach to the problem of weight management that has been helpful to the majority of my patients.

I developed the concept of the Draznin Mile, in which the *duration* of activity, rather than the actual distance covered, is the measure of exercise. Later, I added the concept of the Draznin Calorie, in which any serving of food containing 100 calories is counted as one Draznin Calorie.

Using this system and a dozen Draznin rules of lifestyle, eight out of every ten of my patients were able to lose weight, keep it down, and prevent or get rid of their diabetes. This is an 80% success rate!

This is why I am ready to share my approach with millions of people who wish to lose weight and rid themselves of their Type 2 diabetes.

3

Our
Weight
in Numbers

The most amazing fact in the field of weight management is that the overwhelming majority of dieters in the United States do not need to lose weight, yet many people who do not need to lose weight are trying to do so. It is a culturally driven perception of "self-image" that governs a widespread belief that one must be one or two clothing sizes smaller than one actually is. In contrast, only a small number of significantly overweight people are on diets.

This sounds like a paradox. Shouldn't it be the other way around? Shouldn't overweight people diet? The fact, however, remains—obese people are seldom on a diet.

However, as we examine this apparent paradox a bit more carefully, we will see the depth of the problem. The discrepancy is easily understood when we learn that 95% of those who lose weight on any diet regain it within the next twelve to twenty-four months. Not surprisingly, they give up. Frustration and denial replace drive and perseverance.

A survey conducted by *Consumer Reports* of the efficacy of various diets revealed that only 3% of the people in the survey had managed to complete formal weight-loss programs in the three years prior to the study. Among those who had finished, the average success rate was only 26%. This is less than a third of the 3% of people who began dieting! Eventually, low self-esteem settles in for the duration, frequently hidden under the cover of bitterness and eccentric defiance. As a group, obese individuals have lower incomes and less education than do nonobese people, and more frequently they remain single. This is the price they pay even before taking into account the adverse health consequences of obesity.

Because most of us in the land of plenty carry an extra layer of subcutaneous fat, the question on everyone's mind is, "How much is too much?" For years, the answer was relatively simple—if your weight is 20% greater than your ideal body weight, you are obese. With an answer like that, one immediately asks the follow-up question, "What is the ideal body weight?"

The first attempt to define the ideal body weight came with the publication in 1959 of the Metropolitan Life Insurance Company tables. At that time, the tables demonstrated that the risk of premature death increased along with increased weight. The desirable weight, according to the Met Life tables, was 126 pounds (57 kg) for a 5-foot 4-inch (1.63 cm) woman, and 154 pounds (70 kg) for a 5-foot 10-inch man (1.78 cm). Today, over 80% of the American public exceed these standards.

If you are a medium-built man or woman, you can approximate or "guesstimate" your ideal body weight. To do this, women should count 100 pounds for the first 5 feet of their height. Then they should add 5 pounds for each inch over 5 feet. For example, a 5-foot 6-inch woman would calculate her ideal body weight as 130 pounds (100 lb for the first 5 feet, and 5 lb × 6 = 30 lb for the additional 6 inches). Medium-built men should count 106 pounds for the first 5 feet, and add 6 pounds for each additional inch over 5 feet.

For example, a reasonable "guesstimate" of the ideal body weight for a 6-foot man is 178 pounds (106 lb for the first 5 feet and 6 lb × 12 = 72 lb for an additional 12 inches). Subsequent studies have shown that a ratio of weight to height (defined as weight in kilograms [kg] divided by the square of the height in meters) is a better surrogate for the risk of death from heart disease. This new ratio came to be known as the *BMI*—Body Mass Index. For those of us who think in pounds and inches, the BMI can be calculated by dividing weight in pounds by height in inches squared, and multiplying the quotient by 703. For example, a man who weighs 200 pounds and is 70 inches tall has a BMI of 29 ($200 \div 70^2 \times 703 = 200 \div 4900 \times 703 = 28.7$ or 29). It was also found that increases in BMI were associated not only with heart disease but with many other health conditions. Today's consensus (not without caveats) is that a BMI greater than 27 confers a progressively increased risk of adverse health consequences (Table 3.1). Obesity is clearly associated with diabetes, hypertension, heart disease, arthritis, and gallbladder disease, as well as cancer of the endometrium, breast, prostate, and colon.

Table 3.1. BMI and the Risk of Death

BMI	Diagnostic Category
19 to 25	Normal weight
26 to 29	Overweight
30 to 35	Obese
35 to 40	Severely obese
Over 40	Morbidly obese

Sex	BMI: Lowest Risk of Death
Men	23.5 to 25
Women	22 to 23.5

Therefore, one way of defining the ideal body weight is to say that only a weight not associated with adverse health consequences is ideal. For practical purposes this would be the weight that yields a BMI of less than 27.

A BMI of 19 to 25 is accepted as normal. Those of us with a BMI between 25 and 29 are considered overweight, and those with a BMI of over 30 are said to be obese. A BMI of 30 to 35 characterizes the moderately obese; a BMI between 35 and 40 defines severely obese people, and those with a BMI of over 40 are morbidly obese.

The first important caveat in using the BMI to define obesity is that some very muscular and athletic people have increased BMIs, with no negative impact on their health risk. That is because their increased weight reflects the weight of strong muscles, and not excess fat.

One of the best examples of the influence of muscle mass on the BMI has been provided by Dr. Gary J. Davis, of Evanston Hospital, in a letter to the editor of the *New England Journal Medicine* (December 30, 1999). Dr. Davis reported that the basketball player Michael Jordan, by many accounts the athlete of the century, has a BMI of 24, being 1.98 meters (m) tall and weighing 95 kg. This BMI places Jordan in the upper end of the healthy-weight group, although his body-fat content is under 10%. Even more striking, the body-fat content of another NBA star, Shaquille O'Neal, is reported to be approximately 5%, but his BMI is 29.7 (2.18 m height and 141 kg weight), placing him clearly in the obese category!

The second caveat is that, at any given BMI, individuals who are less fit have higher health risks than do their well-trained peers. In a study at the University of Alabama, researchers found that unfit, lean men with BMIs of 25 or less had twice the risk of death from all causes than did fit, overweight men with BMIs of 27.8 or greater. Thus, degree of muscle development and state of fitness can greatly influence health risks outside the parameters of the BMI.

Finally, the distribution of fat in either the upper body (apple-shaped obesity) or the lower body (pear-shaped obesity) also confers different health risks, with upper-body obesity being more closely associated with adverse health consequences, such as heart disease, obesity, and hypertension.

Upper-body obesity can be detected easily by measuring the circumference of the waist. The numbers to remember are: waist circumference greater than 40 inches in people younger than forty years of age, and waist circumference greater than 36 inches in those over forty years of age. Individuals with these measurements have significantly increased cardiovascular risk. Around the world, both body weight and the prevalence of obesity are increasing rapidly. Epidemiologists, nutritionists, and diabetologists firmly believe that we now live in an era of epidemic obesity. The Worldwatch Institute, an Internet watchdog group, estimates that worldwide there are more obese than malnourished people. Today, 15% to 20% of European adults and 50% to 55% of Americans are significantly overweight (Table 3.2).

Table 3.2. Prevalence of Obesity

Group	Frequency of Obesity
U.S. adults	55% Overweight
	22% Obese
U. S. children	22% Boys obese
	25% Girls obese
European adults	20% Overweight

Each year, an estimated 300,000 people in the United States die of causes related to obesity and its complications. Conservative estimates of the health-care costs associated with obesity exceed $70 billion annually. The National Health and Nutrition Examination Surveys carried out by the National Center for Health Statistics have shown that 22.5% of the U.S. population is moderately-to-severely obese (have BMIs greater than 30), whereas some 55% of the total population is considered overweight (BMIs greater than 27). This is a startling jump from the 14.1% obesity between 1971 and 1974, and 14.5% between 1976 and 1980. Today, 63% of American men and 55% of American women have BMIs of 25 and higher, indicating that more than half of U.S. adults are considered either overweight or obese.

When the risk of death from all causes together—or from cancer or heart disease, separately—was calculated as a function of weight, it was found to increase substantially throughout the range of moderate-to-severe overweight individuals, both men and women, in all age groups. The lowest risk of death was found in men with BMIs of 23.5 to 25 and women with BMIs of 22 to 23.5. The relative risk of death remained low until the BMI exceeded 27 in men and 25 in women. In people with BMI values greater than these, the relative risk of death increased steadily.

Recently, the AARP (the American Association of Retired Persons) issued a report on the health status of older Americans. It states that, even though "Americans over fifty are living longer, smoking less and developing fewer disabilities, increasing obesity could cancel the health gain." The report also states that, between 1982 and 1999, obesity nearly doubled, among those over age fifty, increasing from 14.4% to 26.7%.

Equally impressive is an increase in the prevalence of obesity among children. In boys aged six through eleven, the percentage of obesity increased from 15.2% to 22.3% between 1963 and 1991, whereas, for girls the percentage of obesity climbed from 15.8% to 22.7%. These numbers were steadily on the rise through the 1990s. Many pediatricians, pediatric endocrinologists, and physicians working with adolescents express genuine concerns about the wave of obesity and even Type 2 diabetes among children and young adults.

The reason or, more appropriately, reasons for this dramatic increase in the prevalence of obesity are not clear, and I cannot offer you a definitive answer. Obesity has a relatively strong genetic predisposition, even though the genes responsible for this specific obesity-prone background have not yet been identified.

However, the rapid development of this epidemic cannot be explained by genetic influence alone. There is no reason to believe that there has been a major recent change in the genetic makeup of inhabitants of the Western world. One can assume that the propensity for obesity, the genes that predispose us to store energy and gain weight, must have been with us for generations. Recent environmental factors must have made a huge impact in order for the incidence of obesity to explode.

Improvement in the general availability of food, particularly of the high-caloric-density items, and a sedentary lifestyle are among the most important changes introduced in the last two to three decades.

I would like to draw your attention to an interesting relationship between the increase in the prevalence of obesity, in the last twelve to fifteen years, and historical changes in nutritional recommendations in the United States. In 1921, it was recommended that we consume 20% of our daily ration in the form of carbohydrate. This figure gradually increased to 40% in the 1950s, and to 45% in the 1970s. In the 1970s and early 1980s, there was a tendency among nutritionists and diabetologists to consider carbohydrates, especially refined sugars, "pure, white, and deadly." Such was the title of the book published by a British diabetologist, Dr. J. Yudkin, in 1986. Since then, the perceptions of nutritionists, and their attitudes toward carbohydrates, have changed dramatically. Suddenly, around 1985 or 1986, American nutritionists began advocating 60% carbohydrate in a healthy diet! What we call the "prudent" diet of the 1990s recommends that the food we eat contain 50% to 55% carbohydrate.

Even though one cannot draw any conclusions about a cause-and-effect relationship, a distinct parallel exists between the jump in carbohydrate consumption and the rise in obesity. Why did the experts in nutrition increase their advocacy for carbohydrates? They did not mean to harm us. They did not wish to worsen the epidemic of obesity in this country. They recommended what they saw as the best strategy, at that time. And yet they have created a monster that will take years to undo.

First of all, most of the well-meaning specialists in nutrition are also committed to strenuous exercise and heavy-duty workouts. They bike and run, and they fill aerobic classes to capacity. They are constantly engaged in recreational activities and proudly display to the rest of us their slim, muscular bodies, dressed in sweat-drenched athletic attire. They need tons of extra energy to cover the expenditure that occurs during exercise, and they find this readily available energy in high-carbohydrate food. They became and remain completely oblivious to the fact that most of us do not exercise at all! They have blanketed us with the message of the benefit of a high-carbohydrate diet, forgetting a simple truth—that sauce for the goose is not always sauce for the gander.

At the same time that nutritionists and exercise-enthusiasts were promoting their love for the high-carbohydrate diet, scientists began to understand that cholesterol and other fats might have a detrimental effect on the heart and blood vessels. At the beginning, no distinction was made between "bad" fat and "good" fat; between the "Western" diet and the "Mediterranean" diet, between the influences of saturated and unsaturated fats. Fat in the diet became synonymous with the death penalty. This grew to the point where some parents withheld milk from their children, in their zeal to eliminate fat from their offspring's diets. The food industry, willingly or unwillingly, was dragged into this craze. "Low fat" and "no fat" items filled the shelves of supermarkets. The problem was that all that "nasty" fat was being replaced by huge amounts of carbohydrates! Elimination of fatty foods and reduction in fat content might have had a beneficial effect, as this would have reduced the total number of calories consumed, but not when all those calories were simply replaced by carbohydrates.

Poor reasoning inadvertently killed the good deed, much like the proverbial road to Hell that is paved with good intentions. Many food items, particularly those that contain hefty doses of carbohydrates, proudly display the "Food Guide Pyramid" on their labels. The base of the pyramid represents bread, cereal, rice and pasta, food choices recommended by the guide. For a sedentary individual, this pyramid is not an ancient wonder, but the best prescription to promote obesity!

Obesity is not a trivial and innocent condition. Approximately 300,000 Americans die every year from complications attributable to obesity. These complications of obesity constitute the second leading cause of preventable death in America, after complications from smoking.

Obesity also contributes enormously to the burden imposed on our society and health-care system by chronic diseases that frequently coexist with obesity. One of the most common of the conditions that accompany obesity is Type 2 diabetes (see Chapter 6 for definition and details). Obviously, not all overweight or even severely obese individuals develop diabetes, but the risk is substantially increased with weight.

Conversely, statistics show that over 85% of patients with Type 2 diabetes are obese. Each year, approximately 800,000 Americans are diagnosed with the condition. About 90% of these, or 720,000, have Type 2 diabetes. If 85% of these newly diagnosed individuals are obese, the country will acquire 612,000 patients with diabetes and obesity annually.

There is a slightly higher proportion of women with diabetes than men, and the incidence of diabetes increases with age. On average, African Americans and Hispanic Americans are almost twice as likely to have diabetes as are Caucasians of similar age. It is estimated that, in the United States, approximately 25% of all adult patients with Type 2 diabetes belong to minority groups. Diabetes contributes to approximately 300,000 deaths per year. The death rate is twice as high among middle-aged people with diabetes as among middle-aged people without diabetes.

For example, the relative risk of heart attack is 50% greater in diabetic men, and 150% greater in diabetic women, than in their nondiabetic counterparts. Diabetic men are 50% more likely to die suddenly (sudden death is mainly due to heart attack or stroke) than men in the general population. In women, the difference is even greater, with sudden death being 300% more common in diabetic women than in nondiabetic ones.

Both obesity and diabetes are closely associated with heart disease, mainly atherosclerotic coronary artery disease, leading to heart attacks, chest pain (angina), and stroke. Problems with atherosclerosis in patients with diabetes and/or obesity begin with what is called "inflammation" in the vessel walls. The marker of this inflammation is the appearance of a protein termed *C-reactive protein* (*CRP*). The greater the inflammatory process, the more CRP is found in the blood. Recent studies have indicated that consumption of food items with a high glycemic index (see Chapter 11 for details) resulted in substantial increases in appearance of CRP in blood in apparently healthy middle-aged women. These findings suggest that intake of food with high concentrations of rapidly absorbed carbohydrates may increase the risk of atherosclerosis and heart disease.

Poorly controlled diabetes triggers numerous other complications and medical problems. In the United States, diabetes is a leading cause of new cases of blindness among people twenty to seventy-five years of age. Almost half of new cases of end-stage kidney failure leading to either dialysis or kidney transplantation are related to diabetes. Most patients with diabetes suffer nerve damage after fifteen to twenty years with the disease. Diabetes is also a leading cause of nontraumatic leg amputations, and approximately 20% of male patients with diabetes complain of impotence.

Finally, the total health-care and related costs of the treatment of diabetes and its complications exceed $100 billion annually. This is larger than the gross national product of many countries in the world. It is not surprising that a problem of such magnitude is on the minds of thousands of Americans who are eager and almost ready to turn the tide of obesity in this country.

C H A P T E R
4

The Law
of Conservation
# of Energy

Despite amazing advances in the biomedical sciences, physicians and scientists do not really know why some of us gain weight so easily, while others eat just about everything they see (the so-called "see-food diet"; you see food, you eat it!) and remain slim. We also have very little information about why some of us overweight creatures develop diabetes, while others, equally overweight, do not. Much of it is most probably genetic, determined by the genes we have inherited from our parents.

The first Draznin rule is: The most important step in life is to choose your parents correctly.

If one were to follow this rule (and it isn't easy!) and did it well, the rest would simply fall into place. One would neither be overweight nor develop diabetes. However, the gene (or genes) that determines our destiny to become overweight is extremely prevalent and occurs with great frequency. It is safe to say that the majority of us, given unlimited access to food, have a tendency to gain weight.

Centuries ago, when the food supply was erratic and predictably unpredictable, the genes that allowed our ancestors to store more fat, and thereby more energy, were beneficial and, as such, spread among the population. Today, in a time of plenty, these genes are more than just a nuisance, and we have to fight their influence on an almost daily basis.

Energy is the most fundamental requirement for all aspects of life. For any biological process to occur, an organism, whether it is a single-cell alga or a complex mammal, must possess enough energy to cover the demands of this process. The very survival of the organism depends on finding and acquiring appropriate quantities of energy to sustain life. However, if an organism acquires more energy than is necessary to cover its needs, excess energy is stored and is used appropriately when the new energy intake is limited.

Let us digress for a moment and examine what determines our ability to accumulate fat. Most of us have heard about the law of conservation of energy (even though just a few of us truly understand it).

$$\text{Energy we consume} = \text{energy we expend} \qquad (1)$$

If we consume more energy than we expend, excess energy will be retained and stored by the body, and the equation will look like this:

$$\text{Energy we consume} - \\ \text{energy we expend} = \text{energy we retain} \qquad (2)$$

The energy we expend consists of three parts: the Basal Metabolic Rate; the energy we expend to support physical activities; and the energy we expend to support miscellaneous functions of the body (we don't really know where it goes). The Basal Metabolic Rate, or BMR (also known as *Resting Energy Expenditure*), is the amount of energy required to support the work of the heart, brain, lungs, and other organs at rest, in the absence of any physical or mental exertion. The BMR accounts for approximately 50% to 65% of our total daily energy expenditure. The energy we expend on physical activity is called *activity thermogenesis*, or *AT* (also known as *Voluntary Energy Expenditure*), while the third component of energy expenditure is known as *NEAT*, *nonexercise-associated thermogenesis*, the amount of energy we spend fidgeting.

Finally, a small amount of energy is spent on breaking down (digesting) and absorbing food, and on the biochemical conversion of nutrients into metabolic intermediates and the production of new energy.

This looks like an investment in a process that generates much more energy in return. This expenditure is called the *thermic effect of food*, or *TE*, and it accounts for about 10% of the total daily energy expenditure. Therefore:

$$\text{Calories}[1] \text{ consumed} = \text{BMR} + \text{AT} + \text{NEAT} + \text{TE} \qquad (3)$$

Again, if we expend less than we consume, the remaining energy will be stored:

---

1. The term "calorie" used in this book represents 1,000 calories or 1 kilocalorie (1 kcal). See Chapter 10 for the scientific definition of "calorie."

$$\text{calories consumed} = \text{BMR} + \text{AT} + \text{NEAT} +$$
$$\text{TE} + \text{calories in storage (weight gain)} \qquad (4)$$

Conversely, if we expend more than we consume, we will lose energy from storage and lose weight:

$$\text{BMR} + \text{AT} + \text{NEAT} + \text{TE} - \text{calories consumed} =$$
$$\text{calories removed from storage (weight loss)} \qquad (5)$$

With food being the only energy source for creatures like us, the mouth is the only loading dock for delivering energy supplies to the body. We know that man does not live by bread alone, and yet his food is his only source of energy. If we expend almost all the energy we consume, very little will be left over to store.

In other words, the energy that remains in the body by the end of the day is the difference between the energy we have obtained from food and the energy we have spent during that day. Roughly, each time the amount of energy consumed exceeds the amount of energy spent by approximately 3,500 calories, we gain a pound (1 lb) of fat.

This means that just a little over 500 calories per day, in extra food, will be converted into a pound of fat, in a week. This equation, 3,500 calories = 1 lb of fat, is important to remember not only because of its negative connotation, but also for your future success in losing weight. A deficit of 3,500 calories will result in a 1-lb weight loss.

The second Draznin rule is:
If longevity is in your genes, the
quality of your life is in your hands.

The law of conservation of energy is indisputable, unshaken by any doubts, and it remains the basis for our understanding of weight gain and weight loss. But the law comes with caveats. Nothing in life is as simple as it appears to be. First, not all the food that enters our mouths is consumed by our bodies and utilized as calories. Some of this food is never absorbed. It passes through the gastrointestinal tract and is expelled at the other end.

For example, let us assume that two individuals, Mr. A. and Mr. B., have each eaten a bowl of cereal containing 300 calories of energy. That day, Mr. A. had diarrhea. We do not know at this point why he received an urgent call to the bathroom. He may just have returned from a trip to a foreign country (traveler's diarrhea), or he may have lactose intolerance, or some other medical problem.

Regardless of the cause of his diarrhea, he will absorb only part of the 300 calories he consumed. He will certainly have consumed fewer calories than Mr. B., who has no gastrointestinal problems.

We should remember, however, that diarrhea and constipation are examples of extreme differences in food absorption, whereas in real life there is a spectrum of degree of food absorption among people. Variations are numerous. Chances are you and your life-partner do not absorb exactly the same numbers of calories, even after eating exactly the same meal.

The second important variable in food absorption is that certain foods are absorbed much better and faster than others. For example, a teaspoon of sugar is absorbed almost instantaneously, whereas a teaspoon of pasta requires significant time for digestion. The complex carbohydrates of pasta must first be broken down into simple sugars, and only then are they absorbed. In contrast, each molecule of table sugar consists of only two simple sugars that are readily absorbed. It is not surprising that we absorb 8 ounces of ice cream much faster than 8 ounces of filet mignon.

Recently, new therapeutic strategies have been developed in an attempt to modulate food absorption, and thereby influence caloric consumption. The class of drugs called *alpha-glucosidase inhibitors* blocks the breakdown of complex carbohydrates into simple sugars. Complex carbohydrates are not absorbed in the small intestine, and they are subsequently moved down through the intestine to be evacuated.

As a result, if you eat a plate of pasta while taking these drugs, only a portion of your serving will be absorbed. A great deal of your pasta will escape breakdown and absorption and will be eliminated. Similarly, a new drug, *orlistat*, blocks the activities of enzymes that help absorb dietary fats. Therefore, when you take orlistat, only a fraction of the dietary fat that found its way into your mouth will be absorbed.

But this tinkering with natural absorption is not without side effects. When carbohydrate-breakdown in the small intestine is impaired, the carbohydrates move to the large intestine, where local microbes have a field day, as they love to decompose these carbohydrates. While the microbes propagate and proliferate, and digest as many carbohydrate molecules as they can find, they also create a lot of gas in the large intestine of the person taking these medications.

Gas has a natural way of escaping, which places this person in an untenable position. Orlistat, we now know, blocks the absorption of fat. This unabsorbed fat is now sliding down into the large intestine, and it may leak out, very often uncontrollably.

These side effects are usually minor and create only minimal inconvenience, but occasionally they can push a person into social isolation.

Not only do absorption and consumption of calories differ among individuals, but, once these calories are absorbed, their utilization can be very different from person to person. Let us return to our friends Mr. A. and Mr. B. Mr. A.'s diarrhea is now over, and he and his friend, Mr. B., each eat two slices of pizza; at about 700 calories per piece, for a total of 1,400 calories.

By the time they finish, it is about 10 P.M. Mr. A. and Mr. B. are equally physically active. They both go to sleep. Their bodies use the newly acquired energy to support their breathing, food digestion, heart and brain activity, urine production (all these organs work, even as they sleep), and occasional movement during sleep (turning and tossing in bed). Their bodies expend a sizable amount of energy to cover their basic metabolic needs, the so-called Basal Metabolic Rate, or BMR. It turns out that, because of differences in their genetic makeup, these two gentlemen have very different BMRs. Metabolically speaking, Mr. A.'s body is extremely efficient. He requires half the energy that Mr. B. requires to support his metabolic needs. While he is asleep, his body uses only 800 calories, leaving 600 calories (1,400 calories – 800 calories = 600 calories) for storage and future use.

In contrast, Mr. B.'s body is exceptionally inefficient, and he has had to use 1,100 calories to support his basic metabolic needs. This means that he has only 300 calories left for storage and future use (1,400 calories – 1,100 calories = 300 calories).

Not surprisingly, Mr. B. will not gain as much weight as Mr. A., even though they both ate exactly the same amount. When they wake up and go to the local "Y" to work out, they will discover an interesting detail. In the absence of physical activity, Mr. A. burns fewer calories than does Mr. B. Therefore, Mr. A. will have to exercise almost twice as much as Mr. B., in order to reduce to the same degree the amount of energy he stores.

There is one more thing that Mr. A. and Mr. B. (and the rest of us) should know about their "individualized" ways of utilizing calories. The way these calories are directed to either storage or utilization is under the constant and rigorous control of *insulin*, a hormone responsible for the maintenance of normal levels of glucose in the blood.

The activity and the amounts of this hormone, and its ability to work, are critically important for the utilization of glucose by muscles and fat, for energy storage in both the liver and in muscle, and for the growth and development of new and old fat cells in the body.

The latter is particularly important to understand. One cannot accumulate fat and become overweight in the absence of insulin. People who develop insulin deficiency, so-called Type I diabetes, lose weight very rapidly, in a process called *lipolysis*, which is an accelerated breakdown of fat cells. We will return to insulin later in this book, but for now it will suffice to say that both the levels and the activity of insulin represent the third important variable that modifies the law of conservation of energy in the human body.

The Draznin Mile: A New Concept of Exercise

I t is no secret that most of us do not like to exercise. Hence,

The Third Draznin Rule is:
Desire to exercise is
inversely proportional to age.

Healthy preschoolers, almost without exception, are remarkably active. Chasing your three- or four-year-old offspring can be an exhausting full-time job. By the end of grade school, however, the vast majority of children stop running, skipping, and jumping. The average child in an American family now spends three hours a day in front of the TV set, and at least one-and-a-half hours a day in front of the computer. In junior high school, a physical education hour is considered boring by at least 75% of students. At the same time, four basic food groups emerge as the staple diet of teenagers:

- Fast food
- Soft drinks
- Candy
- Sugar-coated cereals

By the age of thirty, only a tiny minority of individuals engage in regular exercise. For those over thirty, sport is now a spectacle—something we view from a chair, a sofa, or bleachers. At the age of forty, we enter a controversial period of life known as "middle age." (By the way, "middle age" is best defined as your own age, dear reader, and younger.)

In addition to the plethora of well-described peculiarities attributed to middle-age crises, many middle-aged men and women make a feeble attempt to return to an active lifestyle. This attempt is almost never successful, and rarely lasts longer than a year. A notable exception is good tennis players. Tennis players stay active longer, usually until their knees can no longer take the abuse. Golfers, particularly those who drive electric carts, indulge in self-deception.

The truth of the matter is that, unlike competitive sport, where the goal is to be first (by definition—the strongest and the best), exercise for the sake of sweating, in the name of longevity, is simply contrary to human nature. It is much more pleasant to lie by the pool with a good book in your hands (after a quick five- to ten-minute dip) than to swim multiple laps for an hour.

Over 80% of houses in my neighborhood have a basketball hoop. In the last five years I have not seen a single neighbor over forty shooting hoops! I have seen a few of my forty-plus neighbors jog. But the grimaces on their faces as they return home reveal both the misery and the displeasure caused by this form of exercise.

Recently, biking, particularly family bicycling, has come into vogue. For a while, it was very encouraging to see a family of four or five on a bike path, but it appears that most people give up biking as a form of exercise as soon as their teenage children stop riding with them.

Having said all this, I wish to proclaim that exercise is the single most important element for living a healthy life. The right amount of physical activity makes us feel better, helps keep weight down, supports our aging backs, allows for better circulation, and beefs up our ability to cope with stress. The question is, how can we incorporate the right amount of exercise into our lives; into our daily routines? How can exercise become one of the basic activities of daily living, such as bathing, dressing, eating, and so forth? If we who have an inherited aversion to exercise could only find a way of making exercise an integral part of our lives, we would lose weight, reduce blood pressure, remove at least 80% of our tension and anxiety, defeat diabetes, live longer, and feel better.

Years of searching for the "magic formula" have finally paid off with the discovery of the "Draznin Mile." Here is my formula—you walk three to four Draznin Miles each day, or you jog three Draznin Miles every other day. The Draznin Mile is the simplest way to measure your exercise. Here's how it works: The Draznin Mile defines the duration of your exercise, not the distance and, certainly, not the speed. Ten minutes of jogging or twenty minutes of walking equals one Draznin Mile. If you have jogged for ten minutes, you can call it a mile. If you have jogged for twenty minutes, you have done two miles, no matter what the actual distance was. The distance is totally irrelevant. Never, never, never worry about the distance. *The time is what is important.*

If it so happens that you have, indeed, jogged one mile in ten minutes, you are doing much better than expected. A ten-minute mile means that you can cover six miles in an hour. Please, never even think of doing that! You don't need it. No one needs it. All you need to do is three Draznin Miles, meaning a thirty-minute jog. If your weight is 175 pounds, with a jogging speed of ten minutes per mile, you will burn 11 calories per minute, or 330 calories in thirty minutes.

Do you see how easy it gets? If you jog two Draznin Miles, you burn 220 calories. In real life, however, for ordinary people like you and me the speed is totally irrelevant. Thus,

The fourth Draznin rule is:
A ten-minute jog covers one
mile and burns 110 calories.

I recommend that you jog at least three Draznin Miles every other day. Doing that, you will burn 330 calories every other day, or about 1,000 to 1,200 calories per week.

Two things I want you to keep in mind, however. The first is the intensity of exercise. It is not important at all when you first embark on my program. At the beginning, the most important point is to engrave a habit of exercising firmly into your daily life. At this stage, the critical element of my program is to incorporate physical activity into a new lifestyle. Later on, the intensity will become a significant issue to consider.

Low-intensity exercise is basically equivalent to the Basal Metabolic Rate, BMR, in terms of energy expenditure. This is why gardening and cooking do not help in losing weight. One is active, all right, but the intensity of the activity is too low to burn excess energy.

The intensity of exercise must be at least moderate so as to expend energy over and above the BMR. Exercise physiologists call this "exercise at 65% or 75% of maximal capacity, determined by your heart rate and oxygen consumption." I can assure you, however, that, if you do three Draznin Miles a day, at least five days a week, you will reach the necessary intensity to achieve your goal.

The second thing to keep in mind is your gender. I guess that rarely escapes our minds. What I really mean is that there is a significant gender-dependent difference in energy expenditure, particularly at the tender age of fifty-five and over. In order to burn 300 calories, a sixty-five-year-old man must exercise for approximately forty minutes. In contrast, a sixty-five-year old woman must exercise for seventy minutes to burn the same 300 calories. Whether or not this difference is related to loss of estrogen function during menopause is unknown, but the fact remains—women must exercise longer, at the same level of intensity, to burn the same number of calories as men do.

Now, what if you cannot jog? Not to worry. This is just fine. The Draznin walking mile is what you cover during a twenty-minute walk. In other words, if you have walked for twenty minutes, you have covered a mile. Your actual speed (if you indeed were to cover one mile in twenty minutes) would be three miles per hour, or half a mile in ten minutes. At that speed, you burn 5.55 calories per minute.

But, as with jogging, the actual distance is irrelevant. The Draznin Mile is a twenty-minute walk. Thus, if you walk for forty minutes, you have done two Draznin walking-miles, and burned 220 calories. Not bad! After a sixty-minute walk, you will have lost 330 calories.

The fifth Draznin rule is: A twenty-minute walk covers one mile and burns 110 calories.
● ●

It is easy to see that, if you jog or walk a Draznin Mile (ten or twenty minutes, respectively), you will lose approximately 110 calories.

I recommend that you walk for sixty minutes, at least five days a week. You can do it in one walk, or split it into two sessions: a walk in the morning and one in the evening. Your goal is to do three Draznin Miles every other day, if you are a jogger, or three to four Draznin Miles every day, if you prefer to walk.

Then, when you talk with your friends or relatives or colleagues, you should proudly say that you are doing three or four Draznin Miles either every day or every other day. They will be duly impressed, and you will truly be doing a great favor for yourself.

This is your goal, but you should start on a much smaller scale. Common sense never hurts. As far as I am concerned, common sense dictates starting with a short five-minute walk. Just stroll out of your house and walk for five minutes along the straightest segment of the road in front of your dwelling. Walk five minutes by your watch.

That would certainly mean that you would need another five minutes to return home. So take a deep breath, and continue toward home. Congratulations! You have just done a ten-minute walk and covered 0.5 Draznin Mile.

If you cannot walk for five minutes in each direction, you have a serious problem, and this book is unlikely to help, at this stage.

Remember that your goal is to walk three to four Draznin Miles. You are not that far off. By the second week you should increase the time you walk in each direction to ten minutes, for a total of twenty minutes of walking—and that is a Draznin Mile! This is what you should do for the entire week.

You should increase the time you walk by two minutes per week, and, five weeks later, you will be walking two Draznin Miles a day, or twenty minutes, equal to one Draznin Mile, in each direction. Do that for an entire month. Do not skip a single day. I want you to do a month of two Draznin Miles per day. In so doing, you will expend 220 calories a day in addition to your normal daily energy expenditure.

At the end of the month you will have two options. You can continue increasing your walking time (and distance) by two minutes a week, until you are doing three Draznin Miles per day, or you can start walking in the evening (before or after dinner), and build your evening walk up to one or two Draznin Miles.

Some of my patients have honestly complained, and not without reason, that walking is inordinately boring. Fifteen or twenty minutes might be okay, but anything beyond twenty to twenty-five minutes becomes a difficult chore. Fortunately, electronic engineers have invented the "Walkman," the "Discman," and other listening devices that are exceptionally helpful in this regard. Just tune in your favorite radio program and begin your march. Instead of listening from your couch to the click and clack of National Public Radio, put on your earphones and go for an hour's walk while still enjoying your favorite recording artist or composer. You will find that the boredom of walking will vanish with the first musical chords. I even have patients who listen to books on tape while walking. I just hope this does not replace their reading hour!

By the way, if you decide to use a treadmill at home, you should consider placing it in front of a TV set. Most of my patients watch TV at least thirty minutes a day, being addicted to the local and national news and various news-related programs. I recommend that they do it while walking a couple of Draznin Miles, and many do. I must admit—I do it myself! If you opt for jogging, and have never exercised before, you should start with a two-minute jog each way. Even though it sounds like nothing, that is the best way to get into this routine. As with walking, you should add two minutes of jogging in each direction every week until you are jogging three Draznin Miles comfortably, every other day. Congratulations, once again—you have reached your goal!

Before we end this chapter, however, there is one more point to discuss. One day I spent a full hour outlining an exercise program for a patient, Mrs. J., only to learn, at the end of our conversation, that she cannot walk! She has had frequent dislocations of her ankle and cannot really undertake the risk of daily walking.

Thus, we had to turn to alternatives. The first alternative is swimming. It is a lovely form of exercise, for good swimmers. Unfortunately, I have found that, for most of us, it is not a good option. There is not enough muscular work in leisurely, noncompetitive swimming. Most people get tired because of breathing long before their muscles have expended sufficient amounts of energy. But if swimming is your only option, a twenty-minute swim equals one Draznin Mile. Three Draznin Miles every other day is all you need!

The second alternative is bicycling. This form of exercise is much better, but one must use a stationary bike and not a street bike. Not all of us feel comfortable on a street bike; this is true not only on the street, but even along bike paths. As a rule, people who are significantly overweight do not have the agility necessary to ride a bike. Finally, bike riding carries an inherent danger of falling, which is better avoided.

The problem with either a street bike or a stationary one is that riding without resistance is very inefficient in terms of burning energy. One has to spend much more time on a bike to achieve the level of energy expenditure that one would attain per unit of time jogging. Therefore, if you must be on a bike, thirty minutes of nonstop pedaling without resistance equals one Draznin Mile. To do three Draznin Miles, you will have to pedal for ninety minutes. However, that can be rather boring. One can increase the effectiveness of bicycling by choosing programs with either more resistance or doing uphill rides. In any event, biking can be a viable alternative to jogging or walking (Table 5.1).

Table 5.1. Draznin Mile Equivalents

One Draznin Mile equals

1. 10 min jogging or
2. 20 min walking or
3. 20 min swimming or
4. 30 min biking without resistance,
   and burns approximately 110 calories.

Three Draznin Miles a day will allow one to burn 330 calories.

A word of caution is needed for those who are actually preparing to buy new walking shoes. Everyone who is over the age of thirty-five or who might have other medical conditions, particularly known heart problems, must undergo a stress test before embarking on an exercise program. Your primary-care physician should refer you to a specialist to perform this test. This is a simple but extremely important precaution that should not be overlooked.

People who have already developed complications of diabetes should be extremely careful with their exercise regimen. This is particularly true for those with diabetic retinopathy (problems with the blood vessels at the back of the eye), kidney disease, and those with heart conditions. They should not be doing weight lifting, jogging, or boxing. Walking and swimming are the most appropriate forms of exercise for these individuals. Assuming you have no problems, within four to six months you should make three Draznin Miles your daily routine.

Insulin, Production and Storage of Energy, and Regulation of Weight

I believe a little dose of science is in order at this point. I subscribe to a theory that the more people understand about their medical conditions and the ways their bodies work, the greater the chances for successful therapeutic interventions. This is particularly applicable to the health problems that require lifestyle changes.

Having said this, I acknowledge readily that not everyone is interested in the science underlying his or her medical problems. I would not be affronted at all if you decide to skip this chapter entirely or return to it later, after finishing the rest of the book (I hope you'll do the latter). This chapter is written to make this scientific background available to those who wish to learn more about insulin, energy, and regulation of weight.

Insulin is undoubtedly one of the most important hormones in the human body. Without insulin, people do not survive more than just a couple of weeks; seldom as long as a couple of months. This condition of complete, or almost complete, lack of insulin is known as Type 1 *diabetes mellitus*. Insulin is the only hormone in the body that reduces blood sugar levels. It

- Is produced in the pancreas
- Is released in response to meals
- Stimulates utilization and storage of sugars
- Stimulates formation of new fat and proteins
- Prevents breakdown of fat and proteins, and
- Is absolutely required for survival

Type 1 diabetes most commonly occurs in children and young adults (hence, it was formerly known as "juvenile onset diabetes"), but it can appear at any age. It is believed to be an autoimmune disease, wherein an unknown trigger commands the body to destroy its own insulin-producing cells. Insulin is a life-saving treatment for patients with Type 1 diabetes. Insulin is a protein produced in the pancreas, a gland located in the upper part of the abdomen, and is released into the bloodstream in response to sugar.

When we ingest carbohydrates, they are broken down into simple sugars, mainly glucose, as they pass through the small intestine. Glucose is then absorbed into the bloodstream, and this glucose-enriched blood flows immediately around the pancreas, stimulating the release of insulin. Even though other factors also contribute to the release of insulin, the rule of thumb is that the more sugar we consume, the greater the amount of insulin is released to help utilize this sugar.

Utilization of glucose generally means two things: to produce energy to support bodily functions, and to store excess glucose for future use. The body is amazingly efficient in this process. It will utilize only what it needs to cover its energy expenditure. Whatever is left over (please recall the law of conservation of energy!) will be stored under the watchful eye of insulin.

This excess glucose can be stored in two ways. First, molecules of glucose can be linked together, forming a glucose-storage depot, called *glycogen*. Second, when the glycogen stores are fully replete, the remaining molecules of glucose can be coverted into fat that is going to be stored in fat tissue. It would be okay to store energy today for tomorrow's use; for a rainy day, so to speak. The problem is, in the land of plenty, this rainy day doesn't arrive. We continue to consume food and, therefore, energy in excess of our needs on a daily basis. As we consume more and more beyond what we can expend, insulin will gladly do its job—stimulate the storage of more and more glucose and fat in the body.

Glucose is stored in the liver and in the muscle, but fat . . . oh, boy, don't we know where it is stored!

The sixth Draznin rule is: What doesn't kill makes fat!

This is actually an old South African proverb, conveyed to me by a colleague, an excellent endocrinologist and a South African native, Dr. Mervyn Lifschitz. I have adopted this saying as an important rule. Insulin is a life-saving hormone for people with Type 1 diabetes, but in everyone else it helps produce fat! Luckily, there is at least one way to minimize the damage. One should and, actually, one must, limit the amounts of carbohydrates, especially pure, refined sugars, in the diet. If less sugar reaches the pancreas, less insulin will be released, and less energy will be stored as either glycogen or fat.

In contrast to patients with Type 1 diabetes who suffer from insulin deficiency, some people with diabetes have enough insulin but it just doesn't work properly. These people require greater amounts of insulin to achieve normal utilization of glucose by their organs and tissues. These individuals are said to have an "insulin resistance."

In other words, their ability to utilize glucose as an energy source in response to insulin is reduced. Therefore, they require additional output of insulin to maintain normal levels of sugar in the blood. At some point, these patients fail to produce enough insulin to achieve this goal and they develop what is known as Type 2 diabetes mellitus (Table 6.1).

Table 6.1. Two Types of Diabetes

Type 1

Usually an autoimmune destruction of pancreatic beta cells with a resultant insulin deficiency. Frequently begins in childhood and in young adults, and insulin treatment is mandatory for survival. Approximately 10% of all patients with diabetes have Type 1 diabetes.

Type 2

The cause of this most common form of diabetes is unknown. It frequently begins in adulthood, primarily in individuals who are overweight. It is characterized by inefficient action of insulin (insulin resistance) and inadequate insulin release. Approximately 90% of all patients with diabetes have Type 2 diabetes.

The fact that insulin is needed to ensure normal utilization of glucose is well known to the public. What is much
less known, and remains almost unappreciated, is what
insulin does in the metabolism of proteins and fats. Without insulin, proteins in muscle break down into individual
amino acids, weakening the musculoskeletal system.

At the same time, stored fats break down into individual fatty acids and leak out, melting, as it were. A
person with a complete lack of insulin rapidly loses
weight as a result of the accelerated breakdown of proteins and fats.

Overall, the truth of the matter is that, without
insulin, fat cells will not develop, and those cells that have
been developed previously will lose their fat! In other
words, none of us would be able to gain fat mass in the
absence of insulin. Conversely, we can only increase our
weight if we have sufficient amounts of insulin in our
circulation.

Even though insulin is critically important, it is not
the only hormone involved in the regulation of weight.
Several other hormones and chemical substances in the
body help regulate appetite, satiety, and weight maintenance. These include leptin, neuropeptide Y, melanocor-
tins, Ghrelin, and orexins A and B, to name a few. Their
presence and their influence also indicate that our expectations of finding a single medicine that will cure obesity
in all overweight individuals may not be realistic. There
are simply too many factors that influence our ability to
gain, lose, and maintain weight. Instead, interventions
directed at multiple targets in the complex world of energy balance may be more appropriate and are likely to
be much more successful.

Signals of satiety and hunger and of thinness and
fatness are brought to the brain from the peripheral tis-

sues, after being generated in the stomach, liver, gut, pancreas, and fat cells. A very specific area of the brain, a small region known as the *hypothalamus*, has been recognized for some time as the area of the brain responsible for both satiety and eating behavior. In the hypothalamus, signals arriving from the periphery are being processed and integrated in various brain centers. The molecules that participate in this process are called *neurotransmitters*, as they transmit appropriate information from one brain center to another.

One of the most important signals is transmitted by a neurotransmitter known as *serotonin*. Several lines of experimental evidence suggest that serotonin induces early satiety. Based on this evidence, compounds that stimulate serotonin action have been advocated for the treatment of obesity. For example, a famous (or notorious) combination of *phentermine* (phen) and *fenfluramine* (fen) was found to be extremely effective in suppressing appetite; unfortunately, it was also associated with adverse effects that led to its withdrawal from the market.

Overall, it is not unreasonable to foresee that, in ten to twenty years, physicians should have at their disposal medications that will be able to influence appetite, satiety, and eating habits significantly. These new pharmacological agents will, effectively, change both our body weight and our body composition.

For the time being, however, the best approach is to embrace the Draznin rules. The dietary modifications described in this book and the Draznin Mile are your best bets for losing weight and maintaining your desired weight.

Let us now return for a brief moment to the Basal Metabolic Rate (BMR), the amount of energy required to support body functions at rest: for example, while we sleep or thumb leisurely through the pages of the local newspaper.

The more energy we use, as the BMR, to support the work of our hearts, lungs, brains and the like, the less energy will remain in our energy stores. As always, the energy we use for the needs of our resting bodies is derived from food. If food is not consumed, either intentionally (as, for example, during an overnight fast, or during an attempt to lose weight) or unintentionally (if one is starving, as a result of either food deprivation or another disease), the energy to provide for the basic functions of the body is mobilized from the energy stores. This energy is initially derived from glycogen (carbohydrates stored in the liver and in muscle), which runs out fairly quickly, and then from fat (stored as fat tissue), which lasts longer.

Now that we know that the energy to support the life of the organism is derived from foodstuffs, let us briefly review how that actually happens. How does my slice of pecan pie convert into the energy I spend moving from the sofa to the refrigerator?

Dr. Hans Krebs, a scientist who received a Nobel Prize in 1953 for his discoveries of the major steps in the biochemistry of energy production, elegantly divided this process into three stages. Thanks to food labels, everyone now knows that the items we consume are composed of three major nutrients (as we call them, "macronutrients"): proteins, carbohydrates, and fats. In the first stage of energy production from food, large molecules are broken down into smaller units. Proteins are reduced to amino acids; large carbohydrates are converted into simple sugars, such as glucose; and fats are broken down into glycerol and fatty acids. Even though no energy is generated, at this point, this is the critical preparatory step, as only these simple molecules can be used to generate energy at stages two and three.

Certain medications that we use to prevent weight gain or ameliorate diabetes work specifically at this stage. For example, a medication called *Acarbose* interferes with the breakdown of complex carbohydrates into simple sugars, thereby retarding and diminishing the absorption of carbohydrates into the bloodstream.

In the second stage, as these small molecules enter various cells, most of them are further reduced or degraded into a very few simple units that enter the *mitochrondia*—the energy-making factories of the cells of our bodies. Although some tissues, such as heart tissue, prefer using fatty acids to generate energy, in most cells of the human organism a healthy competition exists between fatty acids and glucose for the privilege of being burnt for the sake of producing new cellular energy.

Stage three is the real factory for production of energy. Remnants of sugars and fats are burnt in the energy-producing furnace to generate energy that is stored in high-energy compounds, *a*denosine *tri*phosphate, abbreviated ATP. The ATP molecules function like a battery, supporting the life of each cell in the body.

Carbohydrates, the most abundant source of calories in the human diet, are present in both plant and animal products, and they are easily broken down into simple sugars for speedy absorption. Carbohydrates are an excellent source of quick energy, with 1 gram (g) of carbohydrate providing 4 calories. Excess carbohydrate is readily stored in the liver and muscles in a form of glycogen that is also easily broken down into single molecules of glucose for quick utilization.

Proteins are built from twenty-two amino acids, eight of which can only be obtained from food. Because these eight amino acids cannot be produced in our bodies, they are termed "essential." The richest source of protein is meat, which, in combination with milk, cheese, and eggs, provides all eight essential amino acids. Many plant foods also contain substantial amounts of protein. Although, like carbohydrates, a gram of protein provides approximately 4 calories, proteins are rarely used to cover energy needs. They are much more suitable as building materials, to create new proteins in muscle, and everywhere else.

Fat is the most significant metabolic fuel we have. One gram of fat provides 9 calories, twice as many as carbohydrates or proteins. Therefore, in terms of acquisition of energy, fat is the most efficient source. It is particularly important for tissues that use great quantities of energy in their work. These tissues are skeletal muscle and heart muscle. For absorption, dietary fats are broken down into single fatty acids and glycerol. In the bloodstream, they travel throughout the body and are either used as a source of energy or deposited in storage, in fat tissue. Approximately 85% of the body's energy is stored as fat.

How is this relevant to what, and how much, we eat? How is it related to our ultimate weight? Or to our ability to lose weight? The answers are complex, but they are directly and critically relevant to the regulation of body weight. According to the law of conservation of energy, if we are to maintain our weight, the energy we generate during these three stages must be equal to the energy we expend. If we generate more energy than we expend, we gain weight. If we expend more energy than we generate, we lose weight. We also have to eat a well-balanced diet so as to avoid unhealthy competition between the macronutrients. If the diet is not hypocaloric, the nutrient that is consumed in excess, whether it is fat or carbohydrate, will immediately be placed into storage.

Despite competition, for most body cells it is easiest to use glucose as a source of energy. Glucose is the most readily available source of energy. This simple carbohydrate is critical for providing energy to the brain, the muscles, the liver, the kidneys, and virtually every organ and every cell in the body. As a source of energy, glucose can be utilized immediately, to generate energy, or it can be placed into storage, as *glycogen*, a chain of molecules of glucose kept together by chemical bonds. When we fast or exercise, glycogen breaks down, releasing individual molecules of glucose into the energy-production pathway.

Unlike plants, animals cannot produce glucose from fat directly. Practically speaking, this means that consumption of a diet with a high fat content cannot raise the blood-sugar levels directly.

In contrast to the production of glucose from fat, the opposite process—the production of fat from glucose—is very much possible in the animal kingdom. After all, bees make fat (wax) from sugar (honey). Piglets grow into large fat pigs and ducklings grow into succulent fat ducks on a carbohydrate-rich diet. This happens because the storage of excess energy in fat is much more efficient than the storage of energy as glycogen (carbohydrates).

In the human, however, this concept has been difficult to prove. Numerous studies have shown only minimal conversion of glucose into fat in human beings. However, in the Central African country of Cameroon, the Guru Walla tribe has an interesting tradition of overfeeding. Guru Walla adolescent boys consume about 7,000 calories in carbohydrates daily, and they gain 12 kg (over 26 lb) in ten weeks, while ingesting only a minimal amount of fat.

Let us now consider the story of Mr. G. Mr. G. is a forty-two-year-old accountant who eats a well-balanced diet, consuming approximately 3,200 calories daily. He does not watch the distribution of fats and carbohydrates in his diet, but he looks for "no cholesterol" items in his favorite grocery store. He leads a fairly sedentary life-style, and his walking is limited to the distance from his car to either his office or a grocery store. His BMI (Body Mass Index) is 29, and his caloric expenditure is approximately 2,800 calories per day. He is concerned with a recently accelerated weight gain.

Discussion. Clearly, as long as his caloric intake (3,200 calories) exceeds his caloric expenditure (2,800 calories), Mr. G. will continue to gain weight. He is said to be in a positive calorie balance (+400 calories), and he will not lose weight, no matter what the composition of his diet is.

At his yearly physical, Mr. G. was found to have cholesterol levels of 290 mg/dl. He began a low-fat diet. He is now buying low-fat yogurt and low-fat cream cheese, he eats pasta twice a day, and he snacks on apples and oranges, consuming about four fruit servings each day. His caloric intake is now down to 2,900 calories. After an initial loss of 3 pounds, his weight had remained stable for four months, but, over the next six months, Mr. G. gained 6 pounds. His cholesterol came down to 260 mg/dl.

Discussion. With the best of intentions, Mr. G. replaced calories derived from fat with calories from carbohydrates. His lifestyle did not change, and his diet is still not hypocaloric (low calorie). Even though he burns carbohydrates, he consumes so many carbohydrates that, in the absence of exercise, the carbohydrate excess is directed to storage and conversion to fat. He would derive greater benefit from this diet if he were to start an exercise program to stimulate his muscles to burn the excess carbohydrates. With Mr. G.'s current lifestyle, a high carbohydrate diet would lead to a greater weight gain and would not help him with his cholesterol.

Mr. G. has read about an "all you can eat," high-protein–high-fat–low-carbohydrate diet. His co-worker lost 10 pounds in three weeks on this new wonder diet. Mr. G. eagerly jumped onto the bandwagon. He now eats three egg omelets and two servings of meat a day, and a lot of cheese, and he drinks a glass of whole milk with each meal. His daily caloric intake is 3,000 calories. After an initial loss of 7 pounds over the first month, he maintained his weight for three months and gained 9 pounds over the next nine months. He has frequent morning headaches, and he is very tired by the end of the day. His lifestyle has not changed.

Discussion. Because he stopped consuming carbohydrates, Mr. G. quickly depleted his carbohydrate storage (glycogen) and lost a lot of water that was stored along with the glycogen. This explains his initial weight loss. Mr. G.'s diet is still not hypocaloric. With his glycogen stores depleted, his liver cannot generate sufficient amounts of glucose after an overnight fast. Because glucose, the main energy source for his brain, is now scarce, his liver makes ketones, a chemical product that can be used as a replacement fuel. However, ketones, when produced in excess, can be toxic. With this compensatory ketosis (a state of excessive production of ketones), Mr. G. began experi-

encing morning headaches, and he is becoming exces-
sively tired by the end of the day. In fact, he is so tired
that he cannot even think about adding exercise to his
daily routine. Mr. G. persists in his mistake of not switch-
ing to a hypocaloric diet. Instead, he is currently on a
ketogenic diet that worsens his fatigue and introduces a
new problem, morning headaches.

Commonsense Conclusions

What Mr. G. should be doing is quite obvious. He must
begin a well-balanced hypocaloric diet and change his
sedentary lifestyle. He should consume a daily diet of
approximately 2,300 calories, with 40% to 45% carbohydrates, 35% to 40% fat (mainly monounsaturated and
polyunsaturated), and a healthy mix of low carbohydrate
and Mediterranean diets.

At the same time, he should start a walking program, building his tolerance to three Draznin Miles a day.
This will assure slow but steady and substantial weight
loss, an improvement in his lipid profile, and, most important, a lifelong weight maintenance plan based on the
Draznin rules of a healthy lifestyle.

A Person Does Not Lose Weight by Diet Alone

Mr. K., whom we met earlier, is sitting in front of me, awaiting recommendations. I see in his eyes, that, in his mind, he has already made a commitment to follow my advice. After much trial and error, he wants to give my program a good try. But is Mr. K. a candidate for a low carbohydrate diet? Would he lose weight, improve his blood sugar level, and lower his blood pressure? Would he reverse his insulin resistance? Would he reduce his risk of developing heart problems and diabetic complications? Would he benefit from a low carbohydrate diet? Would he stick with a "Draznin Mile" program, at home and at work, while on a business trip or on vacation?

These were the questions that crossed my mind as I listened to Mr. K.'s complaints, carefully examined him, and perused his two-inch-thick medical record, while sorting out my approach to his problems.

We are looking at one another, straight into each other's eyes. We are now teammates. We have established a common goal: to defeat his obesity and diabetes before they defeat him.

I know what he has to do, but I also know that progress will be difficult for him. To change a life-long set of habits is not a trivial task. With his commitment before us, I accept him on my team. I make a counter-commitment to him. I will guide him to success. I will be available to him whenever he needs me, and I will use my time and knowledge to lead him to what has now become our common goal.

Every single day, I see patients like Mr. K. in my office. I learned a long time ago that patients without *patience* do not do well. The road to success is filled with frustration and setbacks. I can only promise to do my best to guide them through the roadblocks. They may follow my guidance, but it is up to them to overcome the setbacks.

National statistics do not lie. They clearly show that almost everyone who starts a weight-loss program loses weight. To lose weight initially has never been a problem. The huge problem is that 90% of dieters regain weight within the first year after an initial weight loss!

Frustrated people try again, and then again and again, only to go through the same routine: initial success, followed by a bounce-back after a few short months. No wonder so many individuals give up trying to diet. It is also not surprising that people jump on every new gimmick, on every new diet, and on every new pill that purports to help.

For many, the yo-yo dieting continues through decades. But their efforts will not be in vain if they embrace the Draznin Rules of lifestyle.

Based on the law of conservation of energy, we can state with confidence that, if Mr. K. consumes fewer calories than he expends, he will lose weight. Plain and simple. No miracles. That is why all diets that restrict food-intake work. Physicians and nutritionists call these diets "hypocaloric diets."

"Hypocaloric" means that the diet provides fewer calories than are needed to cover daily energy requirements. While on these diets, patients take in less energy than they expend. They are said to be "in negative energy balance."

In fact, they have to mobilize additional energy from the storage places—that is, from fat and from glycogen (remember, glycogen is the storage form of sugar)—to meet their energy needs. Spending more than one has leads to a loss, whether in money or in extra pounds of flesh. Hence, one would invariably lose weight on a hypocaloric diet.

The easiest analogy to help understand the concept of the negative energy balance is your weekly financial balance. Suppose you receive a weekly salary of $500. Even though you have a savings account in your local bank, you are trying to live from check to check, with a weekly budget of $500. Generally speaking, you spend $500 a week for food, housing, car expenses, and other miscellaneous items. If, one week, you have suddenly spent your $500 by Wednesday, the only way you can meet your financial obligations on Thursday and Friday is by withdrawing additional funds from your savings account. You have just found yourself in negative balance. You can exist in negative balance until you deplete your savings account.

Fat around your waist and hips is your energy saving. If you consume less energy than you spend, you will be continuously depleting your fat storage. Unlike the money in the above example, which we wish would grow monthly if not daily, your goal is to deplete your energy savings and get rid of your fat. Thus, the first thing in Mr. K.'s new lifestyle program is quite clear. Mr. K. must be put on a hypocaloric diet. But what exactly is "a hypocaloric diet"?

If you consume precisely the same amount of energy as you spend, you are said to exist on an "isocaloric diet." In other words, you are in a state of equilibrium, as far as energy is concerned. In this state of equilibrium, you are not going to lose or gain any weight. With the goal of losing weight, what you really wish to know is how much less intake than that of your isocaloric diet you must adopt in order to place yourself in negative caloric balance.

The most scientific way to calculate by how much the diet should be restricted is to measure the Basic Metabolic Rate (BMR) of the person, and recommend a diet that gives him or her 300 to 500 calories less than the BMR.

If we had measured the BMR of Mr. K., we would have learned that his BMR was approximately 2,200 calories. After subtracting 400 calories, we would recommend that he consume an 1,800-calorie diet. For him, this number of calories would be hypocaloric. For most people, a diet containing 1,200 to 1,500 calories is hypocaloric, relative to their BMRs, and they should lose weight while on such a diet.

Some people begin their dieting with a Very Low Calorie Diet, a diet containing between 400 and 600 calories daily. This is a drastically reduced caloric intake, and one would certainly lose weight on such a low caloric intake. However, these diets can be dangerous for people with other medical problems, or even for otherwise healthy individuals. Therefore, one should consult a doctor before starting such a diet. Even with a physician's blessing, no one should be on one of these Very Low Calorie Diets for longer than ten to fourteen days.

All successful diets are hypocaloric, including every popular diet that you can find on the shelf of your favorite bookstore. Whether you are on the Atkins diet, the Ornish diet, the Zone diet, Draznin's dietary principles (after reading this book), or any other diet, you will only lose weight if you consume fewer calories than you expend.

Using the Food Process Nutrition and Fitness Software, version 7.20 (Salem, OR: ESHA Research, 1998), one can easily calculate the caloric content of the popular diets from the menus they recommend.

It turns out that the Introductory Menu of Dr. Atkins contains 1,400 calories per day (including 29 g of saturated fat!). The Zone diet recommends 1,340 calories per day, and the Sugar Busters! Diet recommends 1,000 calories per day.

Absolutely, undoubtedly, surely, and unequivocally, one will lose weight on any one of these diets! Short-term success is guaranteed for those who adhere to these diets. If all these diets are hypocaloric, meaning that you eat less, how come some of these diets tell you "Eat as much as you want, and you will still lose weight." Do they lie?

Not necessarily. But they certainly don't tell you all the truth and nothing but the truth. They play tricks with your appetite. For example, if you are on Dr. Atkins' diet and consume only proteins and fat, your liver will generate a lot of ketone bodies to supply energy to your brain in order to substitute for the missing glucose.

Ketone bodies suppress appetite. However, they can also cause headaches, reduce your ability to concentrate, and make you feel more tired. As a result, you will eat less. Beyond that, a diet of only meat and eggs, day after day after day, doesn't taste that great either. How many strips of bacon and fried eggs can you eat?

You will definitely eat less. At least for a while. Don't forget that, with a complete lack of carbohydrates, you are no longer providing good-quality energy for your brain!

The most problematic issue with the Atkins diet is that we don't really know what kind of damage this diet can do to our hearts, if we manage to stick with it over the long haul. Dr. Atkins honestly believes that no harm will be done by his diet even if it is consumed for many, many years. In fact, he argues that, in the long run, his diet reduces blood cholesterol levels.

I believe that Dr. Atkins is only partially correct. His diet may result in lower production of very low density lipoproteins (VLDL), circulating fats that contain 80% triglycerides and 20% cholesterol. A 50% reduction in VLDL production will result in approximately 10% reduction in cholesterol (50% of 20% = 10%). However, unlimited consumption of saturated fat can be extremely detrimental to the heart and blood vessels, even when cholesterol levels are reduced.

A diet completely devoid of carbohydrates can, and frequently does, cause constipation. Fatigue and nausea may be associated with the ketotic state. Many patients on low carbohydrate diets experience dizziness, and they may have a significant drop in blood pressure when they stand up quickly. A high protein diet also creates an additional workload for the kidneys, and this could precipitate kidney stones and gout.

Overall, until good clinical studies are conducted, it would be prudent to avoid the Atkins diet as a long-term solution. Dr. Ornish's diet is truly hypocaloric. It eliminates fat and many proteins, essentially all food items with high caloric density. You are advised to eat grains and fibers.

Two major problems arise with this diet. First, it just doesn't taste good. After a while, all these wonderful grains, without a trace of fat, appear tasteless. No matter how you slice it, this is not an appealing, palatable diet. At least, not to most of us. Consequently, it would take an incredible commitment on the part of a patient to adopt the Ornish diet as a long-term solution to his or her needs.

The second problem is that, if one sticks to this regimen, one is almost constantly hungry. Not only is this diet hypocaloric, but also its high carbohydrate content constantly stimulates the release of insulin. Insulin lowers blood glucose levels and stimulates appetite. People on this diet are always hungry and are always munching on granola and other grains that provide only short-term relief. It is both masochistic and heroic to stay on this diet beyond several weeks.

The Zone diet is more balanced than either the Atkins diet or the Ornish diet. But it also must be hypocaloric to be successful. While allowing intake of all three major nutrients—protein, fat, and carbohydrate—it limits the overall size of your meal, the size of your meat and fish (no larger than the size of your palm), and the amount of carbohydrates. To stay "in the Zone," so-to-speak, and not be hungry, one has to consume great quantities of low-caloric fruits and vegetables, in other words, roughage.

The Zone diet also has a set of complicated rules that one must follow in order to calculate protein requirements based on several tables and charts. One must also calculate the amount of protein and fat eaten when consuming carbohydrates in order to remain in "the Zone."

In summary, life-long converts to the Zone diet are hard to find. If all these popular diets result in weight loss, how come we, as a nation, are becoming more and more obese? The answer is simple. Nine out of ten dieters, regardless of the regimen they choose, cannot keep up their dietary efforts for long, and certainly not forever. Thus,

The seventh Draznin rule is: A person does not lose weight by diet alone.

Successful dietary modifications must be accompanied by permanent changes in lifestyle, and by exercise. Statistically speaking, the only dieters who are able to maintain their reduced weight are those who incorporate exercise into their lives.

After you have lost weight and shed those unwanted pounds, exercise is the key to success in keeping your body from regaining what you had to work so hard to lose. Let me explain why it is so vitally important.

Today, when the tastiest and the most appealing food items contain both carbohydrates and fat, we overeat without even noticing it. Our energy reservoirs are constantly filled to capacity. The fat we consume is stored as fat, under the skin and inside our bodies, wrapping around our organs, such as the heart, liver, kidney, and so forth.

Fat is our long-term reservoir of energy. It takes time to build up fat deposits and, unfortunately, it takes even longer to get rid of excess fat.

In contrast, for its immediate needs, the body uses energy stored as glycogen, a form of stored carbohydrates. Glycogen is very easily and rapidly made from glucose, in the liver and in muscles. This process is called *glycogenesis*, and it is under the tight control of insulin.

After a meal, complex and not-so-complex carbohydrates are split into individual molecules of glucose, in the gut (intestines). These molecules are then absorbed into the bloodstream and trigger the release of insulin. Insulin pushes glucose into cells and tissues, and it stimulates the deposition of the excess glucose as glycogen in the liver and muscles (the liver picks up glucose without help of insulin).

Thus, our old friend, insulin, helps build up glycogen stores and prevents glycogen breakdown. In contrast, between meals or during exercise, when the levels of insulin are lowest, glycogen is broken down to provide glucose for the brain and other organs. During fasting or exercise, the levels of insulin are low and cannot prevent glycogen breakdown into individual molecules of glucose, which can now be used as a rapidly accessible energy source by all the organs of the body. Hence, glycogen provides energy for the immediate needs of the organism. When glycogen depots (that is how scientists call glycogen storage) are depleted, but the body still needs energy, then and only then do fat cells begin to release fat to provide the required energy.

What is even more important to understand is the opposite process. When the glycogen depots are completely filled, and yet one continues to consume carbohydrates, where do these carbohydrates go? With energy-production not in demand, and the energy stores filled to capacity, the glucose excess is converted to fat.

It is also clear that, if we deplete the glycogen stores, we will have to draw the energy from fat, the only reservoir of energy left.

These glycogen stores can be depleted in two ways. One way is to eat a low-calorie, low-carbohydrate diet, so that insulin will not be able to convert glucose into glycogen.

Another way to diminish our glycogen stores is to exercise. Exercise requires energy and stimulates the breakdown of glycogen so as to liberate the molecules of glucose that can be now utilized in the energy-production pipeline. In the absence of glycogen, and with a low carbohydrate diet, the body will start using fat as the energy source, thereby helping maintain the reduced weight.

Knowing how difficult it is to stay on a hypocaloric, low-carbohydrate diet, it is not surprising to realize that, without exercise, we will almost undoubtedly fail any dietary regimen, and regain all those dreaded pounds. Study after study has clearly shown that only people who accepted exercise as a new way of life were able to keep their weight down, years after shedding the extra pounds.

For quite a long time, patients with diabetes and their physicians have realized that exercise lowers patients' blood-sugar levels. This observation was subsequently translated into valuable practical advice, given to many patients with diabetes. At the same time scientists working in the fields of weight regulation and diabetes wished to know the mechanism of the effect of exercise on blood-sugar levels.

Scientists are very curious people. Not only do they wish to know that action *A* produces effect *B*, but they also wish to learn as much as possible, and understand what happens at every step along the way from *A* to *B*. How exercise helps maintain reduced weight and decrease blood sugar levels is not a trivial question. Better understanding of the cellular and biochemical events accompanying exercise might (and probably will) lead to better treatment options in the future.

Some of the very first experiments with exercise revealed that uptake of glucose by muscle cells can be activated by muscle contractions (which is the essence of exercise!) independently of insulin. Even in insulin-resistant patients—those who did not respond well to insulin—exercise effectively stimulated the entry of glucose into cells, thereby reducing the levels of sugar in the blood.

Thus, exercise was found to be able to circumvent the inactivity of insulin and promote the entrance of glucose from the bloodstream into various organs and tissues. What proved to be especially important for patients with diabetes was that, in response to exercise training, their bodies became much more sensitive to insulin. In other words, insulin began working much more efficiently in those insulin-resistant patients who became involved in a long-term exercise program.

Clearly, exercised muscle demands more energy than does muscle at rest. Energy for cellular utilization is produced mainly from glucose, either from new glucose molecules that enter the cell, or from glucose stored in the cell and liberated from glycogen, a compound that stores glucose. If one exercises long enough, one begins depleting glycogen stores in order to supply glucose for sufficient production of energy.

Freeing up space in the glycogen store is important in at least two ways. First, with a decline in supplies of intracellular glucose, cells begin using fatty acids as an alternative fuel to produce energy. Fatty acids are derived from fat that breaks down to liberate this alternative fuel.

Second, when, some time after exercise, a person consumes carbohydrates, newly absorbed glucose can be deposited in now-depleted stores, and will not be turned away to be converted into fat.

From a practical point of view, exercise is a superb adjunct to both a weight-treatment program and a diabetes-treatment plan. In and of itself, without an appropriate diet, exercise may not be very successful, and certainly is not expected to be curative. But, along with diet and medications (as needed), it helps in keeping weight down and controlling diabetes.

The opposite is also true. Without a meaningful exercise program, diet alone usually fails, and the treatment of diabetes is not very successful. Finally, please remember that the three Draznin Miles a day will make all the difference!

CHAPTER
8

A Tale of
Two Brothers

Do you remember how many times your parents told you that your brother behaved better, studied harder, and kept his room much cleaner than you did? They repeatedly pointed out that he even liked homemade soup, when all you wanted was a slice of cheese pizza. By the time you enrolled in high school, you knew pretty well that your brother, Tom, was very different from you. He was, and still is, a very smart nerd. He could spend an entire evening thumbing through the *Encyclopedia Britannica*, or solving mind-twisters from *Games* magazine.

You, however, with your bountiful energy and awfully short attention span, would rather have played ball, ridden your bike, or played video games. Every time your parents would compare you to your brother, you would scream back, "I'm not Tom! I'm not my brother! I'm Johnny!"

The truth of the matter is that you were absolutely correct. You were, and you still are, very different from your brother. And both of you, Tommy and Johnny, are strikingly different from your parents, distinctly different from your sisters, and a world apart from your cousins.

In fact, no one would ever contemplate comparing you with your cousin, Harry. Everyone in the world realizes that you are not your brother, and that your sister would never be confused with your cousin, Sarah.

Even though we share many genes with, and may physically resemble, other members of our immediate or extended families, we all are individuals, with our own *individual* characters, mind-sets, culinary habits, and athletic abilities.

Why, then, do dietitians and doctors and authors of popular diet books offer one and the same prescription for all of us? Let us now suppose that you and I develop the same disease, hypertension, or high blood pressure. It turns out that you and I live in the same neighborhood, and go to the same doctor, a friendly and knowledgeable family physician. When you and I visit our doctor, we do not expect to be treated in exactly the same way. The doctor is likely to prescribe different medications for us, or, at least, different doses of the same medication.

We realize that, even though we have the same diagnosis, the disease is acting upon two distinct individuals, you and me, causing somewhat different problems, requiring individualized therapy.

Exactly the same principle applies to recommendations with regard to diet and exercise. They simply cannot, and should not, be the same for everyone.

The key is to select the most appropriate regimen for a given patient. Not everyone has to avoid egg yolk, and not everyone must be on chromium and manganese. The amounts of carbohydrate in the diet must be adjusted to the degree of physical activity of the individual person, whereas the amounts of protein must be adjusted according to the ability of kidney to handle the protein load.

Although the goal of a physician who treats many patients is uniform—to achieve the best possible control of blood pressure and sugar levels, and to design the best program for weight maintenance—the means to reach this goal can be as distinct as night and day. The approach and the means ought to be routinely individualized by paying close attention to the patient's state of mind, physical abilities, tastes, habits, work and leisure schedules, and the presence of other medical conditions. Here is a fairly straightforward example of how much different Tom is from his brother, Johnny. *Tom* is a forty-six-year-old self-employed plumber who gets his job-assignments from a general contractor. He is usually out his door at 6 A.M., after drinking a glass of orange juice, and on a construction site forty-five minutes later.

His first meal is about 10 A.M., and lunch is at about 1 or 1:30 P.M. Both meals are usually at the nearest fast-food restaurant. Tom tries to be home before 6 P.M., and he eats dinner with his family at 6:30 or 7 P.M.

Tom is 5 feet 9 inches tall and weighs 190 pounds. His BMI is 28. His weight has been stable for the past five years. Two years ago he developed diabetes that is treated with two pills a day. His fasting blood-sugar levels are still moderately elevated, running at about 150 to 160 mg/dl, except for weekends, when they go up to 200 mg/dl. His cholesterol and triglycerides are also moderately increased.

His brother, *Johnny*, is a forty-nine-year-old clerk with the state Motor Vehicle Department. He eats breakfast at home, at 7 A.M., has lunch in the cafeteria at noon, and dinner at home, at about 6:30 P.M.

At home, Johnny is as sedentary as his brother, mainly watching TV and thumbing through his favorite magazines. However, unlike Tom, who toils on construction sites five days a week, Johnny is sedentary at work as well, spending eight hours at his desk, and occasionally taking a leisurely stroll to the men's room. Johnny is 5 feet 10 inches tall and weighs 215 pounds. His BMI is 31. He has had diabetes for five years, and, despite therapy, his blood-sugar levels constantly hover near and above 200 mg/dl. His lipids are significantly elevated; his blood pressure is mildly elevated.

Discussion: A Tale of Two Brothers. Both Tom and Johnny are overweight and have diabetes. Both brothers have elevated lipids and higher-than-normal blood pressure.

Johnny's BMI is in the "obesity" range, most likely because he leads a much more sedentary life than his younger brother does. Tom is very active during work hours. Neither brother pays much attention to his diet, and Tom's sugar levels are lower because of the vigorous manual labor he is engaged in five days each week.

More severe obesity and higher sugar levels are probably responsible for higher lipids and blood pressure in Johnny. What shall we recommend to Tom and Johnny? If we look solely at the diagnoses, the two brothers appear to have the same disease. One may even assume that they should be treated in an identical manner. This assumption would be incorrect, and far from the reality of the situation.

Tom should start by bringing lunch from home, instead of eating on the go, gobbling hamburgers and pizzas. His daily caloric intake should probably stay about 3,000 calories. I would encourage him to do three Draznin Miles on Saturdays and Sundays, and two Draznin Miles twice a week on weekdays. With just a little more structured exercise and better nutrition, Tom should do very well.

Obviously, adjustments will have to be made if Tom's blood sugar and lipids do not drop to normal levels, despite the changes in diet and exercise. He may need to start taking lipid-lowering medications if his cholesterol remains higher than is optimal for patients with diabetes. In addition, Tom should definitely stop drinking beer on weekends.

Johnny, however, has a much longer way to go to reduce his weight and to improve his diabetes, blood pressure, and lipid levels. His diet should be reduced to approximately 2,200 to 2,500 calories, consisting of no more than 45% carbohydrate, mainly as vegetables, fruit, and fiber.

He must begin an exercise program, building to three Draznin Miles five days a week, as described elsewhere in this book. He would also benefit from behavior-modification, and meditation exercises may help lower his blood pressure. Johnny should start antihypertensive and lipid-lowering therapies right away. Just like his younger brother, he should forget about drinking beer or other alcoholic beverages.

As you can see, despite fairly similar conditions, Tom and Johnny should get individualized therapies even before medications are considered. Their diets may be extremely different, and they should be tailored to their individual tastes and food preferences.

I should add that, after thirty years of practicing medicine, I have not yet seen two identical patients in my examining room, even though some of my patients have been identical twins! I would like to assure you that this is not some sort of "holistic medicine" substituted for traditional medicine. Physicians incorporate individual patient-adjustments into their practices every single day. It is necessary to consider important elements of a patient's life while formulating a thorough assessment and a treatment plan.

However, managed care has increased the pressure to provide low-cost health care, and this prevents some primary care physicians from spending any extra time with their patients to discuss these topics. Doctors are pressured to see more patients in the course of their eight- to ten-hour workdays, and they are not reimbursed for discussing modes of exercise and dietary habits with their patients.

A meaningful discussion of lifestyle modifications cannot be accomplished in five or ten or even thirty minutes. The American Diabetes Association (ADA), a premier health-care organization in this country, issues a yearly compilation of its *Clinical Recommendations*, designed to serve as guidelines for both patients and their physicians, as far as standards of therapy are concerned. These *Recommendations* indicate that, at the time of the initial visit of a patient with diabetes to his or her doctor, the physician must take a comprehensive medical history, perform a meticulous physical examination, collect the details of previous treatment programs, including nutrition, exercise, and self-management education, and obtain information on eating habits, nutritional status, and weight history. At the end of the visit, according to the ADA guidelines, a physician shall formulate both short-

and long-term goals, outline medical and nutritional therapies, discuss lifestyle changes as needed, offer an exercise prescription, and review self-management issues.

If your doctor is doing all this, you are in good hands. Stay with him or her. Unfortunately, this may not happen too often in the primary care setting. Even the best primary care doctors frequently do not have time to accomplish all these tasks. Therefore, to receive this level and quality of care one must see a specialist, an endocrinologist or diabetologist.

Recently, intriguing and revealing statistics from the Third National Health and Nutrition Examination Survey (NHANES III) were published by Dr. Maureen Harris, of the National Institutes of Health. A national sample of 733 adults with Type 2 diabetes demonstrated that 95% of these patients had primary care providers, 88% had two or more physician-visits annually, and 91% had health-care insurance. Moreover, very appropriately, 88% of these patients had been screened for hypertension and 84% for lipid abnormalities.

So far, everything indicated a high quality of care. However, the outcomes of the care were much less satisfactory. Forty-five percent of these adults were obese, with BMI levels of over 30; 58% had poor control of their diabetes, with HbA1C (glycosylated hemoglobin; this represents a measure of glucose control, with values over 6.5% considered abnormal) over 7%; 60% of those with high blood pressure and abnormal lipids were not controlled to accepted levels, and 22% of the patients still smoked cigarettes.

To me, these statistics are very telling. They speak loudly to the fact that primary care physicians do not have time to devote to patient education and to the problems of their patient's lifestyle.

Excellent and dedicated physicians in the primary care practices are at a terrible disadvantage when it cames to the amount of time they can spend with their patients, because the current system of health-care delivery is less than optimal, leaving a lot to be desired. That is why, in the current health-care environment, your family doctor may not be able to direct you properly through the maze of medicinal and dietary choices and other lifestyle-related decisions. Simply put, he or she has no time to do it.

You, however, as a patient or as a consumer, are hungry for this type of information and guidance. That is why you purchased this book and numerous other diet and health guides. You are swimming all alone in this sea of information, searching for a magic lifeboat that will rescue you from the deadly current of your negative lifestyle.

Before we end this chapter I would like to acquaint you with two of my patients, Mr. T. and Ms. E. Both Mr. T. and Ms. E. were significantly overweight, and they had identical BMI levels of 38. But that was where the similarities ended.

Mr. T. was a professor of English literature at the local college, a well-educated man, forty-five years of age, with high blood pressure and gout, and with a long list of psychological problems related to a lack of self-confidence and self-esteem. In contrast, Ms. E. was a twenty-one-year-old single mother of three, with no other health problems, juggling a full-time job in a grocery store with evening classes in a community college, while living under extreme socioeconomic pressure.

The fact that these two patients had identical BMI values had very little to do with the choice of therapy for these individuals. The genetic bases for body size, metabolism, feeding habits, and physical activity—the mechanisms that had caused their obesity, their psychological profiles, their social and economic environment, and their health histories—dictate the selection of therapy.

We are still a long way from complete understanding of how these factors, either individually or in concert, influence weight maintenance and energy balance in a given patient. Sooner or later, you will discover that there is no magic cure-all. There is only knowledge and your own willpower. My book offers you the most honest and commonsense approach to your problems. What more can you ask for?

This book has only one simple goal—to empower you to solve your problems with weight, and, if you have it, with diabetes. This book is based only on scientifically proven facts, contains no gimmicks and no anecdotal information, and reflects my personal experience and the experience of hundreds of my patients who have successfully incorporated the Draznin Plan into their lifestyles.

Treatment of Obesity

Weight loss is all about weight maintenance. Granted, it is difficult to shed extra pounds, but most people can do it over a short period of time. What proves to be exceptionally challenging is keeping the new, reduced weight, and not bouncing back to the pre-diet existence.

How do we treat obesity? How are we going to advise Mr. K., who is so eager to combat his weight problem? What do we say to thousands of others with similar problems? The very first step (Step One) in considering a multitude of therapeutic options is to modify our attitudes toward obesity (Table 9.1). By "our," I mean the attitude of physicians and the attitude of patients.

Table 9.1. Treatment of Obesity

Step One	Modify your attitude toward obesity
Step Two	Set realistic goals
Step Three	Assess your mental readiness
Step Four	Find a knowledgeable and willing physician
Step Five	The Draznin Mile
Step Six	The Draznin Calorie
Step Seven	Modify your eating habits

Before any treatment is applied, society must accept obesity as a chronic health condition, and not as a manifestation of a weak-willed mind. Historically, obese individuals have been considered unmotivated, ugly, and somewhat lazy people, unable to control their voracious appetites.

Ironically, this perception is strongly supported by the numerous diet books that create the impression that losing weight is an easy, simple, and trivial task. These books, according to their authors, offer recipes for losing weight. They imply that the key to losing weight is widely known; it is in your hands, right in front of your very eyes, jumping at you from the pages of the various diet books. The implication is that obese people, those gargantuan monsters, simply lack either interest in losing weight or the willpower to become slim and handsome. Even though the recipe for losing weight is readily available to them, these thankless and thoughtless creatures pass on this wonderful opportunity and simply do not wish to become masters of their own fate.

"I have lost 80 pounds," says a smiling thirty-five-year-old woman, from a full-page testimonial. "You can do it too!"

"I've lost 30 pounds in 30 days!" screams another testimonial. "And I'm *never* hungry!"

Not surprisingly, everyone who believes these statements looks at the obese man or woman with astonishment and with questions. If losing weight is so simple, how come we can't do it?

The truth of the matter is that it is extremely difficult to lose weight. Obese people and those who treat them know better. It isn't simple at all. It should not and cannot be trivialized. Losing weight is profoundly complex and exceedingly difficult.

The treatment of obesity is one of the most frustrating experiences in all of medicine. In many cases, obesity cannot, and will not, be cured. At the present state of clinical and scientific knowledge, it is impossible. It cannot be done, any more than we can attempt to cure diabetes or hypertension. We can improve it, we can control it, and we can certainly ameliorate the health problems associated with obesity, but cure it? I seriously doubt it.

I submit to you that when I hear my patients say, "Doctor, but I cannot exercise!" or " Doctor, I just cannot be on a diet," I do not dismiss these statements lightly. Not all of us can play the violin. Not all of us can draw pretty pictures. Not all of us can throw a baseball (without even mentioning the speed and the strike zone). Why, then, do we expect that all of us should be able to enroll in an exercise class?

Conceivably, because of their genetic makeup, certain individuals "select" to avoid physical activities. Surely, they can be forced to exercise, but of their own volition, they won't. Even if they are fully aware of all the potential benefits of exercise, some people just cannot do it. I would safely bet my nickel that most of us would not continue with violin lessons either.

One can argue that the parallel with the violin lessons is inappropriate, because playing the violin requires talent, while exercising requires only perseverance. Not true. No matter what type of activity you enroll either yourself or your children in, chances are that the majority of the enrollees will drop out within a year, be it a cooking class or a music lesson or a foreign-language club.

We tend to select activities that we enjoy, and therefore are likely to continue with. Thus, for some of us, exercise or a diet could never become an enjoyable part of life. It is always a chore; always a struggle; always a pain. This is precisely the reason for the incredibly high attrition rate from the various diet and exercise programs.

In fact, in one nationwide study, when overweight individuals were offered enrollment in a weight reduction program and were given *free* medications, the attrition rate at the end of a year was a whopping 30%! Thirty percent of people dropped out, despite free medications and special attention to their health care. Truth *is* stranger than fiction.

Recalling that the ideal body weight is the weight associated with the least adverse health consequences, we should aspire to achieve this modest goal, and not to win the swimsuit competition at the local beach club. Thus, the second step (Step Two) in the treatment of obesity is to set realistic goals.

Most experts agree that losing 5% to 15% of the initial body weight is both realistic and achievable. Weight loss of this magnitude also improves many of the health problems associated with being overweight. Some experts in obesity assert that losing 5% to 10% of the initial body weight, and keeping it at that level for one full year, is a commendable goal.

Thus, if Mrs. Q., who tipped the scale at 200 pounds, could lose 20 pounds and maintain herself at 180

pounds for a year, she and her doctor should be congratu-
lated. At that point, the new and slimmer Mrs. Q. and
her physician may set new goals. If, however, she expects
to shed 70 pounds and go down from 200 pounds to 130
pounds she will most likely fail, and will never achieve
her unrealistic expectations.

One should realize that quick fixes to lose weight,
just like get-rich-quick schemes, have never worked, and
never will. Both patients and their physicians should be
well prepared for a long haul, with lifestyle modifications
being the key to their success.

The next step in the treatment of obesity (Step
Three) (please, note we do not use any medications or
any special diets, yet!) is to assess whether or not a patient is mentally ready to initiate serious therapy. And
this state of readiness for a mood and behavioral change
is crucial in an overweight person. If a patient is not ready
to make a major commitment to weight reduction, none
of the programs will work. Because the weight-loss process requires full concentration and sustained effort, it
should not be initiated when other problems, such as family or financial matters, are dominant in a person's life.
This individual will simply fail to devote the necessary
effort and commitment to his or her weight problems
while encumbered with other important concerns.

Not surprisingly, instead of a positive outcome, the
patient will face yet another defeat, with the ensuing
emotional consequences.

Once a patient makes a commitment to change his
or her lifestyle toward defeating obesity, the next step
(Step Four) is to find a physician who has time to deal
with these problems and to guide the patient toward reasonable goals. This is not a trivial task in the era of
HMOs!

People whose BMI levels are under 30 can probably benefit from self-directed diet and exercise programs.
Those with BMIs between 30 and 40 must seek professional guidance, as it is highly unlikely that they will succeed on their own.

My experience tells me that nine out of ten patients
in this weight category will fail to achieve even minimal
success, without appropriate guidance. There are too
many pounds to be lost, too many tricks to be learned,
and too many skills to be applied.

Patients with BMI levels over 40 will most likely
benefit from bariatric surgery, a procedure that surgically
minimizes the size of the stomach and the amount of food
that can be consumed and absorbed.

Self-guided therapy basically consists of careful
attention to diet, eating habits, and exercise. Number one,
numero uno, the key element, the cornerstone of all and
every weight reduction diet is that the diet must be
hypocaloric. If this condition is not met, one might as well
kiss all other efforts goodbye. There will be no miracle,
and one cannot circumvent, overcome, or alter nature's
law of conservation of energy.

If the diet is not hypocaloric, there should be no
doubt that there will be no success and no weight loss.
Thus, if you see or hear an advertisement for a pill that
will help you lose weight while eating anything and everything you wish, don't believe it, even for a second. If you
swallow the bait and decide to waste your money to buy
this "wonder pill," you will be taken for a ride.

Recently, while I was in line to pay for my grocer-
ies, I read an article in one of the popular magazines that
attracted my attention. Written by a dietitian, the article
informed the reader that, if one maintains a diet of 1,400
to 1,600 calories, no food is forbidden, and one can eat

anything and still lose weight, as long as one stays within this range of total caloric intake.

Theoretically, this statement might be true, but, in a practical sense, it is grossly misleading. One simply cannot eat an 800-calorie piece of rich birthday cake in one sitting and maintain a 1,400 calorie diet. One would either eat almost nothing else that day, and remain hungry until the next, or overeat at the next meal (which is exactly what is going to happen!).

The next several steps are bundled together (Steps Five through Seven). They ought to be entertained simultaneously. Each day, one must start eating approximately 500 to 1,000 calories per day less than one expends during that day. Most obese men would lose about a pound a week by consuming around 1,800 calories a day. Most women would lose the same on a 1,400 calorie diet. Losing a pound a week doesn't sound like much, but, multiplying this modest loss by the number of successful weeks, one can expect to lose 26 pounds in half a year, or 52 pounds in a year! This is a very substantial weight loss.

I actually doubt that many of my obese patients can be that successful. At the same time, one should realize that it is very difficult to keep to a nutritionally sound diet on less than 1,200 calories per day. The diet of 1,200 calories or less must be fortified with vitamins and minerals, as described below.

Along with a hypocaloric diet, the patient must embark on an exercise routine, and build up to three Draznin Miles a day, as described elsewhere in the book. The three Draznin Miles must become an integral part of life, like brushing one's teeth, washing one's hands, or combing one's hair. That won't happen in a day, or in a week, or even in a month. But it might happen in a year. That is where commitment to the change comes into play.

The third component of a successful transition to a "leaner life" is the modification of eating habits. In addition to commitment, this one also requires education and knowledge of nutrition. Given a choice, most people in the Western world will select food with 40% fat, up to 20% sugar, and variable amounts of high-glycemic-index[1] food items.

You need to know the reason for changing your long-standing eating habits, how to change them, and what will replace your current habits that are no longer useful. You will have to change when, where, and how you eat.

First, you have to be honest with yourself and carefully write down what you eat, and when you eat it. Then you will identify what you actually wish to change, and can begin working on it, one thing at a time. For example, if you identify that you eat while driving or watching TV, this can be stopped first, before you introduce other modifications. Every week you should have a written plan for your modification goals.

Recently, a telling statement appeared in a review of the influence of dietary composition on energy intake and body weight, written by Drs. Roberts, McCrory, and Saltzman of Tufts University, Boston (*Journal of the American College of Nutrition*, 2002). They wrote, "Although data from comprehensive long-term studies are lacking, published investigations suggest that the previous focus on lowering dietary fat as a means for promoting negative energy balance has led to an underestimation of the potential role of dietary composition in promoting reductions in energy intake and weight loss." In my view this convoluted admission of the fallacy of the past rec-

1. The concept of "glycemic index" is discussed in Chapter 11.

ommendations is an understatement. Clearly, replacement of dietary fat with great quantities of carbohydrates has played a major role in the epidemics of obesity we encounter today.

One way to understand whether eating behavior is important to the prevalence of obesity is to quantify the parameters of human eating behavior. Most commonly, three aspects of eating behavior have been quantified. These are *restraint*, *disinhibition*, and *hunger*.

Dietary restraint is defined as a tendency and ability to conscientiously restrict food intake. This is exactly what the dieters do: they restrict their food intake either to lose weight or to prevent weight gain. This restraint is voluntary, and it relates either to quantity of food or to the type of food one wishes to restrict.

Disinhibition is the tendency to overeat palatable food items either simply in the presence of these items or as a result of other disinhibiting stimuli, most commonly emotional distress. Finally, hunger is a powerful signal for food intake that can easily override voluntary restraint.

Notwithstanding the importance of the interplay between hunger and restraint, higher disinhibition has been shown to be strongly associated with greater weight gain. Because the presence of our favorite dishes before our eyes is one of the most powerful disinhibiting stimuli, it is clearly one of the most important factors in our eating behavior.

Everyone is guilty of this—I'm not sure I can restrain myself when a scoop of chocolate ice cream is placed in front of my eyes. The best way to deal with disinhibition is to avoid buying the high-caloric-density items we have previously enjoyed so much.

Certainly, depression or emotional imbalance can contribute significantly to overeating. Very many people lose control of their eating patterns when they confront their problems at work or at home, or when they slip into depression.

At the same time, you should learn about the energy-values of different food items. You should understand how to evaluate nutrition labels so as to determine the caloric content of the food you consume.

The labels, however, are not as simple as they appear at first glance. They give you the amounts of nutrients in grams (g) in one serving, the serving size, and the percentage of the daily value in a 2,000-calorie diet.

Example: the label of an item you are considering buying tells you that a single serving contains 12 g of fat, and that represents 18% of the recommended daily value.

You must understand that, if you were to eat a 2,000-calorie diet, you could consume 65 g of fat a day (12 g is 18% of 65 g). If you ate this particular item for breakfast, you would have the rest of the day at your disposal to eat the remaining 53 g of allowed fat (65 g – 12 g = 53 g). Sixty-five grams of fat will provide you with 585 calories (65 g × 9 calories/g = 585 calories), which will represent 30% of the 2,000-calorie diet. Even if you memorize grams and percentages for a 2,000-calorie diet, it would be difficult to calculate precisely what you have to eat. And then, if you are placed on a 1,500-calorie diet, all the calculations must be done anew.

Here is a practical example of how you actually do it. Mrs. J. was placed on a 1,500-calorie diet, with the following composition of nutrients: carbohydrates 45%; fat 35%; protein 20%. This meant that she should receive 675 calories from carbohydrates (1,500 calories × 45% = 675 calories), 525 calories from fat (1,500 calories × 35%

= 525 calories), and 300 calories from proteins (1,500 calories × 20% = 300 calories).

Now we have to recall that 1 g of fat yields 9 calories, whereas 1 g of carbohydrates and proteins each yields 4 calories. Upon dividing 675 calories by 4, Mrs. J. will discover that she can eat 168 g of carbohydrates daily. In a similar manner, she will calculate that she can eat 58 g of fat and 75 g of protein.

Armed with this information, Mrs. J. decides to eat for breakfast one serving of food that contains 25 g of carbohydrates, 15 g of fat, and 20 g of protein. She knows that this meal (breakfast) will supply her with 315 calories. She now also knows that, during the rest of the day, she may still eat 143 g of carbohydrates, 43 g of fat, and 55 g of protein. She can now plan very carefully what she will eat for lunch, dinner, and snacks. But, most of all, she realizes that she can follow this diet only if she plans it in advance.

Is that difficult? You tell me. I think it is. At least, it is by no means easy. Can one do it? Can you do it? The answer is "yes," one can, and you can. You don't have to be a rocket scientist, but this is where your commitment and perseverance count.

You will have to write down everything that enters your mouth. You will have to calculate the amounts of macronutrients and the number of calories in every serving you put on your plate. You will have to do that, at least initially, in order to learn what to eat and how much to eat. This learning curve is absolutely critical for your ultimate success.

If you were one of my patients, I would meet with you weekly, or even more often, until your dietary regimen became crystal clear to you. We would go over your dietary recall (a list of the items you eat) and your calculations to ensure you were eating the desired number of calories composed of the desired amounts of carbohydrates, proteins, and fats.

If you are not one of my patients, can you count on the help of a primary care physician? I certainly hope you can, but I wouldn't bet on that. There is nothing wrong with your primary care physicians. I am convinced they are excellent doctors; unfortunately, primary care physicians simply do not have time in their busy daily schedules to devote even ten minutes to these calculations.

They refer their patients to dietitians, who know nutrition and who are excellent in their field, but they do not know your disease. The vicious cycle begins again—patients are left to fend for themselves, perusing the diet books and self-improvement magazines.

And what about diet pills? Do we have a magic bullet that can kill our appetites, melt our fat, and boost our energy expenditure? That would be ideal, wouldn't it? The reality, however, is that such a pill is a long way away. Today, we have nothing like that. Not yet. Such a magic bullet is still a dream for many patients, and for scores of drug companies that would love to offer such a panacea to a "hungry" public.

Currently, only one drug, *Meridia* (sibutramine), is approved by the Food and Drug Administration (FDA) as a long-term therapeutic agent for obesity. Sibutramine works by blocking the reuptake of norepinephrine and serotonin by the nerve cells of the brain. This action of sibutramine results in inhibition of food intake in experimental animals and in humans.

In one well-designed study, patients who took sibutramine lost 8% of their initial weight, as compared with a loss of only 1% to 2% in patients who received placebos (a sugar pill). Most important, the weight loss was still present after twelve months of therapy.

Side effects of sibutramine are usually mild and disappear rapidly, after the drug is discontinued. The most common side effects include dry mouth, headache, constipation, and poor sleep. In many patients, however, physicians have also observed increased heart rate and a mild increase in blood pressure. For these reasons, blood pressure and pulse must be carefully monitored in patients taking sibutramine.

Not surprisingly, sibutramine should not be given to patients with poorly controlled hypertension, irregular heartbeat, or with certain other heart conditions. It should also be used with great caution in patients with glaucoma, in patients with migraine headaches, and in those being treated for depression.

Another way to treat obesity with medications is to attempt to block absorption of fats from the gastrointestinal tract. The idea is that one can eat fatty food and, at the same time, take a pill that will prevent absorption of these fats from the gut (intestines) into the bloodstream. The fat will stay in the gut and will eventually slide down through the loops of the intestine and be evacuated.

Xenical (orlistat) is such a drug. It works by blocking absorption of fat from the gut by as much as 30%. In clinical studies, orlistat produced an average weight loss of 10% of the initial weight, and it was very effective in weight maintenance programs for up to two years with continued use of the medication.

A caveat is that patients taking orlistat should limit the amount of fat in their diets to less than 30%. Otherwise, large amounts of unabsorbed fat will cause oily stools. With so much fat, the stool will slide down the intestine, reaching your undergarment faster than you can reach the nearest toilet! These patients will have an urge to relieve themselves very frequently (called "fecal urgency") and, to their great displeasure, they will not be able to hold it in ("fecal incontinence"). This is a very unpleasant, embarrassing, and annoying side effect, indeed! Limiting the fat content of your diet will help prevent this side effect.

Lately, a great deal of interest has been shown in the potential effectiveness of herbal medications. In particular, a "natural fen-phen" or "herbal fen-phen" has become exceptionally popular among dieters. Most of you probably remember that "fen-phen" was a promising combination of two medications that suppressed appetite. This medical regimen became extremely popular among both physicians and diet-conscious patients. The drugs, however, were found to cause infrequent but severe side effects (such as heart valve problems) and were pulled off the market.

The term "natural" or "herbal" fen-phen refers to a combination of St. John's Wort and Ma Huang, an ephedra herb. When used separately, the former is generally praised for its antidepressant properties, whereas the latter is a mild-to-moderate stimulant. Together, they are reported to be helpful in curbing appetite. No scientific evidence, however, exists to support this claim. Incidentally, herbal remedies are not without hazard. Lately, Ephedra has been under scrutiny for possibly contributing to the death of several prominent athletes who exersized strenuously in the heat of summer while taking this drug.

Finally, one should realize that patients with a BMI greater than 40 who have failed to lose weight with various behavioral and pharmacological approaches should consider surgery as a viable option in treating their obesity.

Today, two types of surgery are usually performed in obese individuals: *gastric restriction* and *gastric bypass.* Gastric restriction is a procedure that creates a small pouch in the stomach that basically restricts the amount of food the stomach can receive, thereby limiting one's caloric intake. Smaller amounts of digested food continue to move along the normal route of the remainder of the gastrointestinal tract.

In the gastric bypass operation, the major part of the stomach and the small intestine are surgically by-passed, thus also reducing absorption of nutrients.

Both procedures, regarded realistically, result in approximately 40% weight loss, with good long-term maintenance. Weight loss, in these patients, is associated with significant improvement in diabetes, hypertension, breathing disorders, and mobility. Surgery, however, is not without complications, and one should select a center that specializes in this type of surgery.

It goes without saying that surgical candidates must be fully informed of potential complications. Many centers require that patients go through a thorough psychiatric evaluation to estimate their strength of commitment and ability to cope. Those of you who are eager to use prescription and over-the-counter medications to fight your weight problems must realize that the long-term safety of these medications is completely unknown.

How long do you believe a medication (even the most benign one) needs to be taken? Will three months suffice? A couple of years? Perhaps twenty years? Will the long-term use of these medications improve or impair patients' health? We simply do not know.

Intuitively, based on common sense and today's scientific information, I would recommend these medications only as a short-term measure, designed to help my patients change their eating habits and their lifestyles. These pills should only lead us to three Draznin Miles a day, and no further.

10

The Draznin Calorie: A Better Way to Diet

Now that we are fully armed with the concept of the Draznin Mile, knowing and accepting that one must log three Draznin Miles a day, we ought to face the second side of the energy-balance equation: the consumption side.

What is the maximum caloric intake we can allow ourselves and still lose weight? What would be a sensible dietary limit that assures weight loss initially, and weight maintenance afterward? And, most important, how can we practically implement such a program over a long period of time, both at home and while visiting friends or eating out?

The answer to all these important questions is the Draznin Calorie. The real "scientific" calorie is defined as the amount of energy needed to raise the temperature of 1 gram (g) of water from 15°C to 16°C (or from 59°F to 61°F). One kilocalorie (or 1 kcal) equals 1,000 calories. The caloric content of food is presented in kilocalories (kcal), so the calories we count in our dietary ration are really thousands of those little units of energy needed to heat a gram of water by one degree. For example, 500 calories consumed or expended are 500,000 calories or 500 kilocalories in "true scientific count."

The Draznin Calorie is quite different from both the chemical calorie and the dietary calorie. The concept of the Draznin Calorie, however, is as simple as the concept of the Draznin Mile. The concept is not difficult to understand, but incredibly difficult to follow.

Every time the body has an energy deficit (that is, we expend more energy than we consume), the brain is bombarded with signals of hunger, prompting the body to increase energy intake—in other words, to eat more. The mind and body work in tandem to maintain the energy balance, and, if possible, to store extra energy for a rainy day. Therefore, the critical question for every dieter is how to comply with a hypocaloric diet, or even with a balanced diet, in order to lose weight or to prevent weight gain.

The first step of my approach is quite obvious. We must eliminate from the diet all items with high caloric density. These are the items that contain a lot of calories per small amount of food—per bite or per gulp, if you wish. These are the food items that contain large quantities of fat or sugar, such as deep-fried food or nondiet soft drinks and juices. These should be eliminated at once.

After eliminating high-fat and high-carbohydrate items from the diet, the remaining food items can be classified as containing between one and six Draznin Calories per serving. Simply look at food labels. They always tell you how many calories per serving the food item contains.

Having this information, you designate any food item that contains fewer than 100 calories per serving as containing one Draznin Calorie.

For example, one egg, one small-to-medium-sized apple, one slice of whole wheat toast, and one glass of skim milk each contain one Draznin Calorie, regardless of the actual calories present. Sound familiar? Remember, when you walk for twenty minutes, you cover one Draznin Mile, regardless of the true distance traveled.

All food items containing between 101 and 200 calories per serving are said to equal two Draznin Calories. Examples include 3 ounces of poultry or lean meat or fish, one dinner roll, or one cup of lean-meat-based soup. Table 10.1 demonstrates the Draznin-Calorie equivalent of the caloric content of food.

Table 10.1. Caloric Content of Food and
Draznin-Calorie Equivalent

Caloric Content	Draznin Calories
Up to 100 calories/serving	1
101–200 calories/serving	2
201–300 calories/serving	3
301–400 calories/serving	4
401–500 calories/serving	5
501–600 calories/serving	6

The eighteen different food items used most commonly by patients adhering to my program are listed in Table 10.2.

Table 10.2. Common Food Items and
Draznin-Calorie Equivalents

No.	Food Item	Draznin Calories
1	1 egg	1
2	2 breakfast turkey links	1
3	1 slice whole wheat or rye toast	1
4	1 glass of skim milk	1
5	3 oz lean meat/poultry/fish	1
6	1 cup vegetables	1
7	1 cup fruit	1
8	1 dinner roll	2
9	1 tsp salad dressing or oil	1
10	1 cup vegetable soup	1
11	1 cup meat-based soup	2
12	1 cup creamy soup	3
13	Appetizer (restaurant)	3
14	Salad (restaurant)	2
15	Entrée-size salad (restaurant)	4
16	Entrée without garnish	3
17	Entrée with garnish	5
18	Dessert	6

The key element of my program is to eat no more than six Draznin Calories per meal, and no more than eighteen Draznin Calories per day. Because one Draznin Calorie equals or is less than 100 calories, consuming six Draznin Calories per meal means that one consumes no more than 600 calories. Consuming eighteen Draznin Calories a day assures that the caloric intake for that day will stay below 1,800 calories. Together with walking three Draznin Miles a day, this would be an excellent and efficient way to lose weight.

By the way, if, at breakfast, you ate only four Draznin Calories, you cannot add the remaining two to your lunch or dinner. Remember that each meal must be no larger than six Draznin Calories. If you eat less, good for you!

The new lean lifestyle is based on spending energy while doing at least three Draznin Miles a day, and consuming no more than eighteen Draznin Calories (no more than 1,800 calories). Many of my patients carry a small pocket-calendar-sized card with the caloric content of allowable food items in Draznin Calories. Simply by checking off the number of Draznin Calories per meal, they can stay within eighteen Draznin Calories a day, and successfully continue with the program.

Table 10.3 provides an example of a breakfast containing fewer than six Draznin Calories.

Table 10.3. Sample Draznin Breakfast

Sample Breakfast Item	Draznin Calories
1 egg	1
2 slices toast	2
1 turkey link	1
1 glass skim milk	1
Total Draznin Calories	5

Restaurant items are more caloric than homemade food. Usually, an appetizer in a restaurant contains 300 to 400 calories, equal to four Draznin Calories. A large entrée-size salad easily contains 400 to 500 calories, and this should be counted as four Draznin Calories. A meat, poultry, or fish entrée, usually larger than 3 ounces, prepared with oils and sauces, and served with garnish, equals five Draznin Calories. Desserts cover the entire meal—six Draznin Calories. Based on this count, when eating out, we have several choices (see Table 10.4).

Table 10.4. Sample Dinner Menus

Choice 1	Draznin Calories
Vegetable soup	1
Dinner salad	2
Entrée without garnish	3
Total Draznin Calories	6

Choice 2	Draznin Calories
Vegetable soup	1
Appetizer	3
1 dinner roll	2
Total Draznin Calories	6

Choice 3	Draznin Calories
Meat-based soup	2
Large entrée salad	4
Total Draznin Calories	6

Choice 4	Draznin Calories
Dessert	6
Total Draznin Calories	6

Choice 5	
Any combination that does not exceed six Draznin Calories	

Dinner at home may contain a plate of salad (one Draznin Calorie) with a teaspoon of no-fat dressing (one Draznin Calorie), a dinner roll (two Draznin Calories) and six ounces of grilled chicken (two Draznin Calories), for a total of six Draznin Calories. One can skip the roll and, instead, have either a larger portion of meat or a side dish of vegetables, still staying within the allowable six Draznin Calories.

With this concept of the Draznin Calorie, the only information you need from the food label is the size of a serving and the number of calories per serving. If the number of calories per serving is under 100 calories, simply count it as one Draznin Calorie. If you decide to eat two servings of this food item, you will consume two Draznin Calories. Make a note on your chart, and make sure you eat no more than six Draznin Calories per meal, and no more than eighteen Draznin Calories per day. I recommend that you keep an accurate record, in Draznin Calories, of what you eat at each meal; do this for three to four months. During this time, you will develop a habit of eating foods with lower caloric density, and in smaller portions. Coupled with a walk of three Draznin Miles a day, you will have developed, and will have learned to maintain, a healthy lifestyle, a slimmer body, and a happier spirit.

Having been so adamant about an individualized approach to my patients' problems throughout this book, I would like to lead you to my practical advice that can serve as the background for your own lifestyle changes. You, or better yet you and your doctor or nutritionist, will be able to modify it, adjust it to your taste, work and eating schedules, family situation, and other health problems you might have. The diet might appear somewhat stringent, but it isn't. There is a great variety of vegetables and grilled fish and meat to satisfy every hue of every taste. Finally, only two requirements stay constant if one wishes to lose weight: (1) one must consume less energy than one expends and (2) three Draznin Miles must complement one's dietary efforts. Here it comes—my Practical Advice.

C H A P T E R

11

Practical
Advice

What about alcohol? What about eating out? What foods should you buy, and how should you prepare meals? What about having a dinner at a friend's house? Do you have to take extra vitamins and/or nutritional supplements? Are there, or will there be, any effects on your prescription and over-the-counter medications? All these are important questions. You must know the answers. And the answers are simple and reasonable, and the advice is easy to follow.

Added Sugars

The term "sugar" is used to designate the *mono-* (single molecule) and disaccharides (two molecules). The monosaccharides are glucose, galactose, and fructose. The disaccharides include sucrose, lactose, and maltose. Many commonly used sweeteners, such as, for example, corn syrup, contain trisaccharides, or even longer molecules of saccharides.

The monosaccharides and disaccharides are also known as *simple sugars*, or *simple carbohydrates*, as opposed to *complex carbohydrates*, which consist of many simple saccharide molecules. Complex carbohydrates must be broken down in the digestive tract before they are absorbed into the bloodstream.

Dietary Guidelines for Americans, published jointly by the U.S. Department of Agriculture and the Department of Health and Human Services, offers a distinction between "added sugars" and the carbohydrates naturally existing in food. Physiologically, however, the body cannot make this distinction and thus treats all sugars, either added or naturally occurring, in the same way. Nevertheless, it is important to understand the term "added sugars" and the impact these sugars have on nutrition.

Added sugars are defined as sugars that are eaten separately or "added" as an ingredient to processed or prepared food items such as soft drinks, ice cream, cakes, and pies. Added sugars include white and brown sugars, maple syrup, corn syrup, honey, molasses, and fructose sweeteners, to name a few.

Consumption of added sugars in the United States has increased steadily, from 27 teaspoons per person per day in 1970, to 32 teaspoons per person per day at the present time, an increase of 23%. Nine specific food items lead the way in presenting added sugars in the American diet: soft drinks (33%), fruit drinks (10%), candy (5%), cakes (5%), ice cream (4%), ready-to-eat cereals

(4%), sugar and honey (4%), cookies and brownies (4%), and syrups and toppings (4%). Soft drinks are the clear winner. Added sugars must be completely eliminated from the diet of anyone who wishes to lose weight.

Glycemic Index

In 1981, a group of investigators led by Dr. David Jenkins proposed to use the *glycemic index* of individual food items in designing an appropriate diet to treat diabetes. The idea was to classify carbohydrate-containing foods numerically, assuming that this might be helpful in treating patients with Type 1 diabetes.

The concept of the "glycemic index" (GI) is fairly simple—each carbohydrate-containing food item causes a rise in blood sugar levels, and the magnitude of this rise, relative to the rise elicited by a pure glucose, becomes the GI of this particular food item. Initial studies by Dr. Jenkins compared changes in blood-sugar levels caused by 50-gram portions of various carbohydrates with those caused by 50 grams of glucose. The higher the rise in blood-sugar levels after a particular carbohydrate, the higher the GI of this carbohydrate.

Later, a 50-gram portion of white bread was used as the standard, instead of glucose. After hundreds of food items were tested (generally in healthy volunteers), it was determined that refined grain products and potatoes have high GI values (causing high elevations in the blood sugar of these volunteers). Legumes and unprocessed grains have moderate GI values, and starchy fruit and vegetables have low values.

During the ensuing twenty-two years, over a hundred scientific studies have been conducted to examine the application of the GI to obesity, diabetes, and even cardiovascular disease. Many popular nutrition books advocate diets based on items with a low GI level. This advice is intuitively correct. If one eats food that causes the least elevations in blood-sugar levels, one would have a lower carbohydrate load, and one should be better able to control one's diabetes.

This concept was later endorsed by the Food and Agriculture Organization of the World Health Organization. In contrast, a typical Western diet contains high concentrations of carbohydrates, because it is based on potatoes, breads, and low-fat cereals.

However, even though the diet based on food items with low GI values makes sense, the concept is not as simple as it first appears, and its utility by no means has a consensus.

First, the GI was determined for each carbohydrate-containing food item—for example, rice, potato, and spaghetti. Most of us, however, eat mixed meals, not just rice or just potato or just spaghetti. We eat chips and fish, meat and potatoes, peanut butter and jelly, pork and beans, and so forth. Most of our meals contain multiple food items. Just look at our soups and gumbos to see how many ingredients are in one plate! The GI of the mixed meal has never been determined.

Second, 90% of the glycemic indices have been determined in experiments with a small number of healthy, young volunteers, who may digest, absorb, and respond to food items very differently from people of middle-age who have certain health problems. And, in fact, many older individuals, and patients with diabetes, digest and absorb food much more slowly than do young and healthy volunteers. Remember that each of us has a unique way of handling food—you are not your brother Tommy!

Third, the GI of a food is influenced profoundly by its type, by its processing, and by its preparation. For example, the GI values of different types of rice varies by almost 100%! Similar differences have been found for different types of pasta, apples, and many other foods.

Methods of food processing, including grinding, pressing, and rolling, affect the GI dramatically. So does the application of heat and moisture, as well as cooling and time of processing. All these steps can damage the outer layers of grains and the chemical composition of starches, thereby affecting significantly the GI of these foods.

Finally, the way a food is cooked also modifies the GI of the food. The amount of heat used, the amounts of water or sauces, the cooking time—all are important factors in modifying the GI of food items. In general, the more we heat, moisturize, grind, or press a starch-containing item, the higher the GI of this item is. And the reason is that warmer, moister, and ground food items are better digested, and more rapidly absorbed.

One can easily drown in the long list of the glycemic indices of many carbohydrate-containing food items published in the International Table of Glycemic Indices in the *American Journal of Clinical Nutrition* in 2002 (the list contains nearly 1,300 data entries), while attempting to design a low GI diet. A better, much more practical solution is to limit carbohydrates in your diet as outlined in my recommendations.

If you want to lose weight, don't complicate your life by trying to identify low-GI food items. Instead, eliminate potatoes, pasta, and all sweet and baked goods from

your diet, and enjoy your carbohydrates in fruit and vegetables, except for bananas, grapes, and corn.

Dietary Fat

There are two types of fat that we consume: cholesterol
and fatty acids. The same cholesterol and fatty acids are
also produced in the body, but consumption of increased
amounts of fat can greatly influence the overall concentrations of fat in the blood and in the bodily stores.

Cholesterol is absorbed from the gastrointestinal
tract with help of bile, which simply functions as a deter-
gent to dissolve cholesterol. After being absorbed, cholesterol moves quickly into the liver, and a large proportion
of it is released back into the gastrointestinal tract.

Because of this efficient recycling, it is very difficult to increase the levels of cholesterol in the blood by
eating additional cholesterol. As a rule, people who have
elevated cholesterol have an elevated production of cholesterol in their bodies.

Other fats, however, are broken down in the gut
(intestines) into single fatty acids. Not all fatty acids are
created equal. They actually come in three varieties: saturated, monounsaturated, and polyunsaturated.

Saturated means that every bond of every carbon
atom in the fatty acid is connected with a different chemical group. When a single carbon atom of the fatty acid
contains an extra available bond, the fatty acid is said to
be *unsaturated*. When more than one unsaturated carbon
atom is present in the molecule, the fatty acid is termed
a *polyunsaturated* fatty acid.

Saturated fatty acids appear to be associated with
heart and blood vessel disease. Unsaturated fatty acids,

especially monounsaturated ones, appear to be protective against cardiovascular disease. Saturated fatty acids (the bad fat) are present in meat, eggs, palm oil, and coconut oil. Polyunsaturated fatty acids are found in cold-water fish, soybeans, nuts, and canola oil. Monounsaturated fatty acids are contained in olive oil, canola oil, avocados, and nuts. The so-called Mediterranean diet is famous for its beneficial effect on the heart and high content of monounsaturated fatty acids.

Alcohol

First off, what do we do with alcohol? To drink or not to drink? For many of us, alcoholic beverages have became a part of life; if not a daily routine, then a social one. To have a beer, a glass of wine, or a cocktail is an integral part of social interactions, whether with our friends, relatives, colleagues, or even alone.

However, if your commitment to losing weight is genuine and serious; if you really, truly want to shed pounds, do not consume alcohol. Each and every gram of alcohol contains 7 calories that will add to your caloric intake. More important, most alcoholic beverages contain a lot of carbohydrates, especially beer, sweet wines, and wine coolers. Therefore, beer and wine coolers are deadly to your diet. Finally, alcoholic beverages increase your appetite. Within minutes after ingestion, alcohol reduces blood-sugar levels and triggers a hunger signal to your brain. With food in front of you, you will inevitably eat more after having a drink or two than you would have with just a glass of seltzer. In patients with diabetes, alcohol may actually raise blood-sugar levels, worsening their control of their diabetes. Because it is so vital to your success, I wish to repeat my advice. If you are serious about your commitment to weight reduction or to a weight maintenance program, avoid alcoholic drinks, by all means.

Having said this, I realize that, on occasion, you may find yourself in a situation where you simply cannot refuse an invitation to imbibe. If you are in such a predicament, and if you find it hard to refuse a drink, I can offer you two options. The first is simply to ask for a glass of dry, nonsweet wine (preferably a red one), and drink no more. Dry table wines contain fewer calories and carbohydrates, and less alcohol content than do other drinks.

As always, with drinking, one should be cognizant of the amount of alcohol consumed. For example, 3 ounces of dry table wine contains 68 calories, whereas a 12-ounce can of beer contains 151 calories. But if you drink 12 ounces of dry table wine, you will consume 272 calories (68 calories × 4 = 272 calories). Similarly, 1.5 ounces of hard liquor contains 107 calories. *Ple-e-ease*, do not drink 10 ounces of hard liquor! Aside from your having consumed 740 calories, your evening may not end well.

Your second option is to ask for a drink that you truly dislike, and just touch it with your lips once or twice during the evening. You will save face, and no one will refill your glass!

Eating Out

When you dine out, follow Draznin rules eight and nine.

The eighth Draznin rule is: If you are overweight and are trying to lose weight, never, ever go to a restaurant that serves Asian food.

The food there might be excellent, but if you have a problem with your weight and/or have diabetes, stay away. Practically all the items on the menu in these restaurants contain sugar, and a lot of it! Not good for a weight reduction diet!

The ninth Draznin rule is: While dining out, order only grilled or broiled meat or fish.

Never order deep-fried, pan-fried, or anything covered with sauces. If you are serious about losing weight, never order pasta, potatoes, or rice, but only green and red vegetables. If your entrée comes with either potato or rice, eat as little as you possibly can, and never more than *half* your serving.

Whenever possible, order an appetizer or a salad, and split an entrée with your companion. When it comes to dessert, fresh fruit is your best option. However, if you have not eaten any carbohydrate at all, choose the least caloric dessert, and split it with your dining partner.

In the restaurant, please talk to your waiter. Ask how large the portion is, and whether you can share your entrée, if it is too big. Find out how the food is prepared—broiled, fried, steamed, or sautéed. Can sauce or dressing be served on the side? Will the chef substitute side dishes?

Don't be shy; waiters love these questions. In their minds, the longer the preorder discussion, the greater the tip at the end of the meal. Conversely, for you the answers can be critical. For example, let us say tonight you fancy clams. Two ounces of steamed clams contain 60 calories, and less than a gram of fat. In contrast, the same 2 ounces of clams—but now breaded and deep-fried—contain 250 calories and 13 grams of fat. Which one should you order?

Now, what do you do if you are invited to someone's house for dinner? If it is a good friend, call the person and share your dietary philosophy. Tell your friends that you can only eat grilled food, and that you are trying to limit both fat and carbohydrate intake. Explain carefully what you mean, and what food you will gladly eat with pleasure and without restrictions. Most people will be very supportive.

If, on the other hand, you do not feel as though you can call and discuss your situation with your host, have a snack at home, about an hour before dinner, so you will not be hungry at the table. When you are not hungry, you are better able to control both your appetite and your choice of foods.

Vitamins and Supplements

Vitamins are absolutely essential for many biochemical reactions within various cells. They actually help numerous enzymes carry on their appropriate functions. Deficiencies in vitamins readily impair these important functions, resulting in malfunctioning of different bodily systems. In extreme cases, vitamin deficiency can cause severe and even fatal disease.

In a similar manner, frequently certain biochemical reactions in various cells require the presence of very specific minerals, such as magnesium, chromium, calcium, and others. Mineral deficiency can also cause significant impairment in bodily functions.

We receive most vitamins and minerals from food. Generally speaking, a normal diet of 2,000 calories or more, which includes meat, dairy products, fruits, and vegetables, contains sufficient vitamins and minerals and rarely if ever requires supplementation. In contrast, however, diets containing 1,200 calories or less do not supply adequate amounts of vitamins and minerals, and these should definitely be supplemented. Similarly, diets that selectively exclude certain food items, such as vegetarian diets or diets without fruits or vegetables, must be supplemented with vitamins and minerals.

Make sure you discuss your needs for vitamins and minerals with your doctor. My practical advice is that you should take vitamin and mineral supplements, particularly iron and folate, if your diet contains fewer than 1,500 calories. If you are a vegetarian, you definitely need vitamins B_2 and B_{12}, as well as calcium, iron, and zinc. If you are over sixty-five, you may need calcium, selenium, and folate. In any event, you must have an informative conversation with your physician about vitamin and mineral supplements.

Choose a multivitamin preparation that provides no more than 100% of the daily value ("% DV" is what is shown on the label) for all the vitamins and minerals included. You certainly do not want any of the side effects of excessive intake of these compounds. Only buy supplements that have the U.S. Pharmacopeia (USP) symbol of quality on their label. Remember that most vitamins are better absorbed with food. However, calcium and iron may decrease the absorption both of each other and of other nutrients. They should be taken separately.

Finally, do not forget antioxidants. Most natural antioxidants are present in dark-green and dark-orange/red fruits and vegetables. The medicinal value of antioxidant vitamins, such as beta-carotene and vitamins C and E, has not been scientifically confirmed.

Prescription and Over-the-Counter Medications

Diets themselves, particularly successful ones, on which the dieter is losing weight, may have an impact on the effectiveness of some medications, and so may certain vitamins and minerals. Also, medications can alter the absorption and function of particular vitamins and minerals. Interactions can go either way, and your medications may suddenly become either more effective or less effective. In both cases adjustments have to be made. That is why you must discuss this issue with your doctor as soon as you begin your dietary efforts.

Cooking and Eating at Home

You can substantially reduce the number of calories you consume by changing your cooking habits, and without sacrificing the taste of your favorite dishes (or at least, sacrificing very little!). The number-one rule is to buy proper ingredients, as described below.

To begin with, the lower the caloric density of the items you buy, the fewer calories will end up on your plate, and, eventually, in your stomach. The second point is to grill, broil, steam, or poach your food, instead of frying it. Here are few other tips that should help you change the way you cook:

- Always trim all the fat from meat, and remove the skin from poultry.
- Always substitute low-fat or nonfat versions of the items in the cooking recipes.
- Serve food from the kitchen, and never bring serving plates to the table. Going for seconds should not be made easy.
- Do not ever watch TV or read while eating. Focus your full attention on the amount of food you are consuming.
- Eat slowly. In fact, eat as slowly as you can. Do not take anything into your mouth until the previous mouthful of food is completely chewed and swallowed.
- Store food out of sight.
- Set aside time to prepare fresh vegetables in bulk, and store them until you use them.
- Do not skip a meal, particularly on a day when you are going to a social function. If you are hungry, you will most definitely overeat.
- Brush your teeth after each meal. The taste of the toothpaste should replace the taste of food.
- Finish your last meal of the day at least three hours before you go to bed.

Grocery Shopping

Here is another critical element of my practical advice: Learn how to select your food in the grocery store.

The tenth Draznin rule is: Never, ever buy any food item that contains more than 6 grams of sugar per serving.

There is only one exception to this rule, and it is milk. Milk is the only allowable fluid that has calories, and the only allowable product that contains more than 10 grams of sugar (actually, 11 g per serving in fat-free milk). The most appropriate food choices should contain no more than 6 grams of sugar, and the best choices should have fewer than 3 grams of sugar.

Items with lower sugar content are there on the shelves; you just have to look for them. You must become a "smart shopper" committed to the Draznin Plan. Let us examine, for example, four Hormel ready-to-eat dinners: Meat Loaf with Tomato Sauce (6 g of saturated fat and 7 g of sugar); Grilled Chicken Breast with Teriyaki Sauce (1 g of saturated fat and 30 g of sugar); Beef Tips with Gravy (2.5 g of saturated fat and 3 g of sugar); and Turkey Breast with Gravy (1 g of saturated fat and 2 g of sugar). It is not too difficult to see which one should be included in the Draznin Plan. The Turkey Breast is the number-one choice, with Beef Tips earning second place.

If yogurt is on your shopping list, you should know that Dannon 99% Fat Free yogurt contains 36 grams of sugar, a Fat Free one has 17 grams of sugar, and the Light'n Fit Creamy yogurt contains only 10 grams of sugar.

When you come to the aisle where you find the English muffins, you will see some with 2 grams of sugar (sourdough), 7 grams of sugar (12-Grain), and 11 grams of sugar (cinnamon and raisin). My choice is clear (the sourdough) and so should yours be. If weight loss is your goal, the Draznin Plan is your best guide to success.

High sugar content is as bad as a high content of saturated fat. *Always read food labels, and never go shopping hungry.* We all know from our very own experience that when we are hungry, we buy food items that we will later regret.

Another suggestion is always go to the market with a shopping list you have prepared at home. If you are driving to the store and discover that you don't have a shopping list, return home and prepare one. With a list, you will buy only what you have preselected—only what you need. Without a list, you will buy on the spur of the moment, usually high-fat, high-carbohydrate items.

As you wander down the aisles examining the shelves, you must understand what the nutrient claims provided by the manufacturers really mean. Table 11.1 offers a partial list for your edification.

Table 11.1. Nutrient Claim and Its Meaning

Term	Meaning
Calorie free	Fewer than 5 calories per serving
Cholesterol free	Fewer than 2 mg of cholesterol per serving and no more than 2 g of saturated fat per serving
Fat free	Fewer than 0.5 g of fat per serving
Sugar free	Fewer than 0.5 g of sugar per serving
Low calorie	No more than 40 calories per serving
Low cholesterol	No more than 20 mg of cholesterol and no more than 2 g of saturated fat per serving

(continued)

Table 11.1. Nutrient Claim and Its Meaning (*continued*)

Low fat	No more than 3 g of fat per serving
Extra lean	No more than 5 g of fat, 2 g of saturated fat, and 95 mg of cholesterol per serving
Lean	Fewer than 10 g of fat, 4.5 g of saturated fat, and 95 mg of cholesterol per serving
Light or lite	One-third fewer calories, or 50% less fat per serving than regular food
Reduced	25% less fat per serving than regular food

As you can see, one must check labels carefully and understand "manufacturer jargon." Many items contain more calories, fat, and sugar than may appear to be the case from reading the label.

Dairy Products

When you shop for dairy foods, remember that they are excellent sources of calcium, vitamin D, and protein. A cup of skim milk, for example, contains 8 grams of protein.

At the same time, there are today many "reduced-fat" dairy products on the market. As a rule, nonfat items have little taste, and many are outright unpleasant. In contrast, low-fat products taste almost as good as do our favorite nonreduced items. Unless you are on a very strict low-fat diet, you should still enjoy low-fat dairy products and not challenge your palate with tasteless nonfat substitutes.

Conversely, if you mix dairy products into recipes (for example, sour cream for salad dressing), the nonfat kinds will do just fine. By the way, instead of buying flavored yogurt, you might try mixing fresh fruit into plain yogurt—do your own flavoring, so to speak. Finally, fruit-containing sorbets are delicious, and they contain almost no fat and no added sugar.

Meat

When shopping for meat, look for the leanest cuts of meat: "loin," "leg," or "round." Also, if you are buying beef, choose the "select" grade over the "choice" grade, as the former is the leaner. Overall, the leanest cuts of beef (when trimmed of fat before cooking) are eye-round, top-round, and sirloin steak. These cuts contain fewer than 7 grams of fat.

The leanest pork cut, with only 4 grams of fat, is pork tenderloin. Trimmed boneless loin roast, boneless sirloin chop, and boneless loin chops contain fewer than 7 grams of fat. In poultry, skinless chicken and turkey are low in fat, with white meat being leaner than dark meat. Always remember that "ground turkey" contains more fat than "ground turkey breast." Duck and goose are much higher in fat than are chicken and turkey.

Soy

Soy, an excellent alternative source of protein, is becoming a mainstream product for many dieters. Soy products like tofu and tempeh take on the flavor of whatever sauce, marinade, or seasoning you decide to use with them.

There are literally hundreds of recipes for the preparation of soy products in many delicious ways.

The main advantage of soy products for a weight-conscious consumer is their low content of both fat and carbohydrates. For example, Mori-Nu Tofu, one of the best-tasting tofus, contains no fat and only a single gram of carbohydrate per 3-ounce serving.

Snacks

Unless you are slim and regularly exercise, avoid all snacks and candy bars. Most commercially available snacks are not high in fat and are not high in carbohydrates, but they represent a mixture of both! Most snacks are low in proteins and low in moisture. They are basically designed for those who need an extra load of carbohydrates between bouts of moderate-to-strenuous exercise. If your goal is to lose weight, the best you can do is to lose any interest in snack bars.

Some people prefer nuts for snacks. Most nuts contain between 8% and 18% protein, and 70% to 90% unsaturated fat. They are usually free of cholesterol. Almonds are rich in calcium and fiber. Chestnuts are unique, because they contain mainly carbohydrate, and they are low in fat. Pecans are among the highest in fat and lowest in protein. Macadamia nuts are sweet and creamy, and they have more fat and calories than do any other nuts. As a rule, an ounce of nuts contains 160 to 200 calories.

Fruit is another popular mid-morning and mid-afternoon snack. Fruit can be fine if it is not overly sweet. Sweet fruit containing large amounts of sugar can cause excessive release of insulin that will, in turn, pre-cipitate the feeling of hunger thirty to sixty minutes after the snack.

Here is a list of food items you should not eat or drink if you are serious about losing weight:

Sugar
Grapes (almost pure sugar—glucose)
Bananas (extremely high carbohydrate content)
Dry fruit (very high sugar content)
Candy
Sugar-coated baked food
Regular soda (a major culprit—high sugar content)
Anything else that contains more than 6 grams of sugar per serving (except milk)
Asian food (unless homemade, without added sugar)
Hamburger or hot-dog buns
Regular bread, rolls, bagels, and pastries
Beer
Sweet wine
Mixed drinks
Pasta
Pizza
Deep-fried food
Breaded meat or fish
Anything else that contains more than 3 grams of satu-rated fat per serving
Sauces (most contain sugar and high amounts of sodium).

Here is a partial list of food items you should mini-mize in your diet:

Low-calorie breads
Dry table wine
Red meat
Potatoes
Rice
Cereals

Rules for eating in restaurants:

- No alcohol
- Meat or fish grilled or broiled only
- Meat portion no larger than the size of your palm
- Never anything fried, deep-fried, or breaded
- Low-calorie sauces and dressing only on the side
- No more than half a portion of the carbohydrate-containing vegetables, such as potatoes or rice
- For dessert (the best choice is to skip it, but you can order it if no carbohydrate-containing vegetables were consumed with your entrée), order frozen yogurt, light fruit pie, or fresh fruit
- Try to have an appetizer, and split the entrée.

As I stated in my introductory letter (Chapter 1), to maintain a diet is not an easy task. In addition to your commitment, the diet must be comprised of items you like to eat and not be too complicated. Finally, without increasing your energy expenditure, you still may fail to lose or maintain your reduced weight. It is the entire package, the Draznin Plan, that you should have in mind when you embark on a journey to change your lifestyle. The rules of appropriate hypocaloric dieting can be summarized as follows:

1. Never eat, buy, or bring home anything that contains more than 6 grams of sugar per serving (milk is the only exception).
2. Never eat, buy, or bring home anything that contains more than 2 grams of saturated fat per serving.
3. Eat no more than six Draznin Calories per meal and no more than eighteen Draznin Calories per day.
4. Do three Draznin Miles a day, to shed extra calories.

Case Studies and a Treatment Plan for Mr. K.

Mrs. Elizabeth E., a forty-eight-year-old self-employed writer, was the mother of two children and had no health problems, except for being overweight and having Type 2 diabetes. Mrs. E. was 5 feet 5 inches tall and weighed 174 pounds. Her BMI was 29.

During her second pregnancy, Mrs. E.'s physician detected elevated blood sugar levels. That was sixteen years before she came to see me. At that time, she was treated with insulin, three premeal injections per day. After delivery, her blood sugar levels normalized, and insulin was discontinued. She did not lose much weight after her pregnancy and, in fact, continued to gain weight over the next five to six years.

Mrs. E. worked from home, and she was extremely disciplined about her writing and editing assignments. She allocated three hours in the morning and three hours in the afternoon to be at her desk. She also spent two hours a day reading. Aside from her usual household chores, she was not involved in any "extracurricular" physical activity.

Eight years earlier, at the age of forty, she had been diagnosed with overt diabetes, Type 2. Mrs. E. was advised to follow a low-fat diet, with 55% to 60% carbohydrates, mainly derived from complex carbohydrates and fiber. She was also started on oral antidiabetic medications.

At that time, Mrs. E. believed it would be easy to adhere to these recommendations, particularly in light of the fact that she had always turned to pasta as a source of healthy carbohydrates, and her entire household loved pasta dishes. Pasta is easy to cook and, with various sauces, provides great variety in taste. But her diabetes remained poorly controlled.

Because Mrs. E.'s blood sugar was continuously above 200 mg/dl and her glycosylated hemoglobin (HbA1C) hovered around 9%, her doctor placed her on two injections of insulin a day. Over the next couple of months, her doctor increased the dose of insulin, and, when Mrs. E. came to see me, she was taking 48 units of insulin in the morning and 36 units before dinner.

Her diabetes improved somewhat, with blood sugar declining to 150 mg/dl and her HbA1C to 8%. However, after that, she gained almost 18 pounds, and that generated in her a lot of anxiety, frustration, and unhappiness.

Mrs. E. realized that, after her insulin injections, she had to eat in order to prevent low blood sugar—the so-called insulin reaction. To deal with weight gain, she began skipping insulin injections, first occasionally, and then on a regular basis.

When she came to see me, she was not taking her insulin on Tuesdays and Thursdays, in an attempt to eat less on those days. She had not disclosed this to her previous physician, and when I examined her, her HbA1C was 9.4%, reflecting almost constantly elevated blood-sugar levels.

Mrs. E., who still did not exercise, decided to increase her physical activity and to spend about two hours a day taking care of her beautiful garden.

Discussion. Mrs. E. was an intelligent woman who had been truly and conscientiously trying to follow the recommendations she had received from her doctor. She wanted to know more about her condition and, for a long time, she adhered faithfully to the prescribed regimen.

It was a failure of the therapeutic program that resulted in her frustration and poor compliance in taking her insulin. Eventually, her fear of gaining weight prevailed over the necessity of controlling her diabetes.

Unfortunately, in this regard, Mrs. E. is not alone. Several major studies have clearly documented significant weight gain in patients receiving insulin to control their diabetes.

Certainly, taking increasing doses of insulin will eventually keep blood-glucose levels in check, but there is a price to pay. And patients pay this price with pounds of gained weight.

I asked Mrs. E. to write down, honestly and meticulously, everything she ate during the next three days. She did, and we reviewed the list of food items that made their way into her diet.

Her dietary recall revealed that she was consuming, on average, 3,100 calories per day. That was clearly too much. To lose weight, she whould have to consume about one-half this amount daily.

We designed a low-carbohydrate diet, with a minimal amount of saturated fat, and reduced cholesterol. She began a hypocaloric diet of 1,600 calories per day. We also reduced her insulin dose by half, and she started a walking program, beginning at twenty minutes, twice a day.

The results were very impressive. Mrs. E. lost 8 pounds in two weeks, her blood-sugar levels decreased to 120 mg/dl, and we further reduced her insulin dose. The plan is for her to stay on her 1,600-calorie diet, build up her exercise tolerance to three Draznin Miles a day, and discontinue insulin. At that time, she may or may not require other antidiabetic medications.

Mr. Frederick D. had a very different problem. He was a forty-two-year-old loan officer with a local bank and had Type 1 diabetes. He was fifteen years old when he was diagnosed. He had been, and still was being, treated with insulin injections, as insulin is the only therapy for patients with Type 1 diabetes. At the time he came to see me, he was administering three insulin injections to himself each day.

Mr. D. had never been advised to keep to a particular diet. Instead, he had been taught to count carbohydrates in his diet, and to adjust his insulin dose accordingly in order to cover his carbohydrate load. He had followed this advice for twenty-seven years. He did it very efficiently, having reached a certain degree of perfection in carbohydrate counting. He could look at his meals and assess the number of carbohydrates almost instantaneously. Then, he would give himself a single unit of insulin for every 12 grams of carbohydrates in his meal. Two years before, he had undergone laser therapy on both eyes, for retinal problems. A year later, he had been found to have an elevated blood pressure of 150/105 mm Hg and had been placed on antihypertensive medication.

A month before he came to see me, laboratory evaluation revealed that his kidney function was significantly impaired. He was told that, within the next three to five years, he would probably require either dialysis or kidney transplantation.

Discussion. Twenty-seven years of diabetes had finally damaged Mr. D.'s eyes and kidneys.

Though laser therapy for eye problems has saved the sight of millions of patients with diabetes, kidney disease remains a grave complication of the disease. Approximately 40% of patients with Type 1 diabetes end up developing kidney failure. Many require dialysis, and many undergo kidney transplantation. Recent advances in the treatment of elevated blood pressure have reduced the rate of kidney failure in patients with diabetes, but it still remains a colossal problem for patients with diabetes, and for the health-care system in general.

Major clinical studies have shown indisputably that better and tighter control of diabetes delays and prevents the development of these complications. Unfortunately, some patients, even with excellent control of their diabetes, can still develop complications.

We do not know why this is, but, conceivably, a certain genetic makeup may predispose these individuals to develop complications.

As for the treatment history of Mr. D.'s diabetes, I strongly disagree with the philosophy of ignoring diet and allowing a youngster to eat everything, and simply take more insulin to cover extra carbohydrates and extra calories. A number of diabetologists, dietitians, and psychologists believe that children and adolescents with diabetes should not be placed on dietary restrictions, as these restrictions may have an adverse psychological effect.

I believe the contrary. Young patients with Type 1 diabetes show tremendous and early psychological maturity. This is true not only for patients with diabetes, but also for young patients with many other serious or chronic illnesses. With appropriate support, these children and young adults would gladly embrace the best approach to their conditions. And my approach to all patients with diabetes is to instill a firm commitment to diet therapy.

Another point of vital importance to Mr. D. was his elevated blood pressure (hypertension). To maintain normal blood pressure is probably the single most important element in the treatment of diabetic patients with even mild hypertension. We now recognize that aggressive treatment of high blood pressure in patients with diabetes prolongs their lives, delays eye and kidney complications, and prevents heart attacks and stroke. A patient with diabetes should never have a blood pressure level greater than 130/85 mm Hg, and, preferably, it should be less than 125/80 mm Hg.

It was imperative for both Mr. D. and his physician to do everything and anything possible to reduce Mr. D.'s blood pressure to desirable levels.

I recommended that Mr. D. eliminate sugar, sweets, and baked goods from his diet immediately. I also designed a diet with low protein, because his kidneys could no longer handle a significant protein load. I would be adjusting his insulin dose weekly so as to find the optimal dose to control his diabetes. The diet was also low in cholesterol and saturated fat.

I began aggressive treatment of his hypertension, with both medications and meditation therapy. Finally, I checked his blood lipid levels and recommended a lipid-lowering medication as well.

Our hope was to delay the progression of his kidney disease, which was still very much an attainable goal, even in the presence of his already-impaired kidney function.

And what about exercise? What about the three Draznin Miles for Mr. D.? At that time, he had to be extremely cautious with his exercise program. Strenuous exercise could further damage his kidney function. I preferred to stabilize his diabetes, to control his blood pressure, and then to have a stress test performed. That would give us a reasonable assessment of the ability of his heart to handle an exercise load. Only at that point would I feel comfortable designing an exercise program for Mr. D.

Now, after we have discussed in detail the role of diet and exercise in weight reduction and weight maintenance, we should be able to give very specific recommendations to many other individuals with obesity and diabetes. I wish to present to you several case studies, examples from my clinical practice, and ask you, the reader, to participate with me in the decision-making process. I want to ensure that you read my book not only for its general educational value but also that you will derive specific information that will be important in helping you address your own concerns with a clearer understanding of them.

The examples I offer to your attention should mirror some of the problems you might have, and they should help you solidify the knowledge you have gained from this book. I hope these case studies will also reinforce the notion that every person is different, and that our advice should be individualized, as much as possible. At the end of this exercise, we will design a very specific program for Mr. Jeffrey K., who is still sitting in my office awaiting answers.

Case No. 1

Jason P., aged twelve, came to see me because of a recent weight gain of approximately 18 pounds. Even though Jason had grown about 4 inches over the previous summer and fall, an 18-pound weight gain rightly alarmed his parents, who brought Jason to my office. Mr. P., Jason's father, was an engineer with a cable company, and Mrs. P. worked as a billing clerk for a group of physicians.

Jason had grown up normally, with minimal medical problems. Over the previous year, he had become very involved with his computer, and now spent almost all his free time in front of his PC. His parents were very proud of his ability to write computer programs and design sophisticated Web pages. They were concerned, however, with his recent weight gain.

For breakfast, Jason usually had a glass of orange juice and a blueberry muffin. He would have a bag of chips and a can of regular Coke at school, and he would eat about two servings of macaroni-and-cheese when he arrived home from school. He would then eat again, at 7 P.M., this time dinner, with his family; the meal usually consisted of chicken with mashed potatoes, or pizza. Jason would drink another can of regular Coke at the dinner table. A large-sized bag of corn chips and a Coke were always present at his computer desk, and he wouldn't even notice how many chips he ate at his computer.

Question. What should Jason do to prevent further weight gain and possibly lose excess weight in the near future?

Answer. Clearly, the computer had consumed Jason to the point that he had neither the time nor the desire to be involved in any physical activity. At the same time, his diet was extremely rich in carbohydrates. On this diet, and without exercise, Jason was about to join the increasing ranks of obese children and young adults.

Before it was too late, his parents should convince Jason (or lead him, by example) to allocate some time in his daily routine for physical activities: walking, biking, playing basketball, swimming; anything but sitting in front of a PC monitor.

Dietary habits would also have to be altered. Muffins, macaroni, pizza, and regular Coke—all must go. Vegetables, fruit, noncaloric drinks, and nonfat meat and poultry would have to be introduced into his diet.

In order to place a twelve-year-old on a diet, all members of the household would have to change their dietary habits. It was absolutely mandatory for Jason to reverse his course toward obesity.

A related question. For which one of the following four twelve-year-olds is a macaroni-and-cheese dinner *not* an appropriate choice?

a. A very active twelve-year-old boy who also plays soccer every day.
b. A normal-weight twelve-year-old boy who spends most of the day in front of his computer.
c. A normal-weight twelve-year-old girl who is a member of a competitive swim team.
d. A normal-weight twelve-year-old girl recovering from surgery for a broken leg.

The answer is **b**. All four children eat an unrestricted diet, making it very likely that the sedentary child who spends most of his day in front of a computer monitor consumes more than he spends. This sedentary youngster will quickly become overweight on a high-carbohydrate and high-fat diet. The girl recovering from surgery will have to adjust her diet when recovery is complete.

Case No. 2

Mrs. Marianne Z., a 5-foot 7-inch woman weighing 185 pounds, worked as a paralegal in a busy law office. She was thirty-five years old and had two children, ages five and seven. She had gained 20 pounds after the birth of her first child, and over 30 pounds during and after her second pregnancy.

   Her thyroid-function tests were normal, and she did not have diabetes. Mrs. Z. loved sweets and pastries, and she prepared a lot of sweet food items for her family. Pancakes with honey, cinnamon rolls, or Belgian waffles were her favorite breakfast foods. She had read that fatty food is bad, and she was trying conscientiously to buy low-fat items. She loved to bake and was proud of her culinary skills. She stayed busy at work and at home, but she was not involved in any structured exercise program.

Question. What should Mrs. Z. do to initiate weight loss?

Answer. The very first thing Mrs. Z. needed to do was to begin a hypocaloric diet. She had to eat less. She had to consume fewer calories than she expended. This was unquestionably the number-one rule for her success.

She had to change the nature of the food she ate, the way she cooked, and the food items she purchased. Many so-called low-fat foods contain excessive amounts of sugar and other carbohydrates that are not good for weight loss. Among her immediate steps, Mrs. Z. had to switch herself and the entire family to noncaloric beverages, change her breakfast routine, and eliminate 90% of her baking.

Without these steps, she would never be successful in losing, or even maintaining, her weight. Subsequently, she would have to find time for three Draznin Miles a day.

A related question. What is the most appropriate breakfast choice for a 5-foot 7-inch woman weighing 185 pounds?

    a. One egg, over easy, one slice of whole wheat
       toast, one unsweetened grapefruit.
    b. One pancake with honey, a glass of orange juice.
    c. One cinnamon roll with marmalade, coffee with
       skim milk.

The answer is **a**. This is the only choice that minimizes the intake of carbohydrates. Choices b and c would fit a high-carbohydrate diet and would be highly inappropriate for an obese woman.

Case No. 3

Mr. Dwayne J. was a forty-two-year-old sales representative who was 6 feet tall and weighed 195 pounds. He traveled extensively within the Western United States, staying in hotels and eating out with his clients and colleagues. During the previous four years, he had gained 25 pounds. He had mild pain in his knees that limited his ability to walk, which he actually liked to do, but for which he could find little time.

Recently, his blood pressure had risen to 140/95 mm Hg. He knew about some "minor" problem with his cholesterol, but he didn't remember what exactly it was. He was otherwise healthy. His father had died of a heart attack at the age of fifty-nine.

Question. What should Mr. J. do to lose weight?

Answer. At he age of forty-two, with elevated blood pressure and, probably, elevated cholesterol, and also a family history of a heart attack, Mr. J. had first to undergo an exercise stress test, and re-evaluate his lipid levels. Provided he was ready for it, Mr. J. ought immediately to start an exercise program, building up to three Draznin Miles a day.

Considering his knee pain, stationary biking or swimming might be his best options. He should also start a hypocaloric diet, eliminating high-fat and high-carbohydrate items from his menu. His new diet should consist of grilled meat and fish, with vegetables. It goes without saying that he should stop drinking alcohol either before or with his meals.

A related question. Which one of these four 195-pound individuals should not eat a 900-calorie shrimp-and-pasta dinner?

a. A 5-foot 11-inch college student competing for a spot on a football team.

b. A 5-foot 7-inch thirty-five-year-old former high school and college wrestler who works out and jogs three miles daily.
c. A 5-foot 9-inch thirty-nine-year-old lawyer who is trying to lose weight.
d. A 6-foot 2-inch, thirty-four-year-old auto mechanic who is on a low-fat diet.

The answer is **c.** A high-carbohydrate meal would not be beneficial to a sedentary person who is trying to lose weight. It might, however, be appropriate for an athletic person who is involved in a regular, more-than-moderate exercise program.

I hope you have answered all these questions correctly. Let us now return to Mr. Jeffrey K., our protagonist and my patient, waiting to hear my advice regarding his weight, diabetes, and high blood pressure.

Without becoming engulfed in many small details, for the purpose of our discussion I submit to you that my advice will be concerned with four general areas: diet, exercise, lifestyle, and medications. Because the "medication" topic is too specific and highly professional, it is clearly beyond the scope of this book. Let us put it aside and discuss my recommendations for diet, exercise, and lifestyle, in great detail.

First there is sensible and realistic hope for Mr. K. Two large, recently completed studies have confirmed what many of us already knew from our individual experiences. Appropriate diet and exercise prevented the development of diabetes in almost 60% of people participating in these studies. In a Finnish study, 172 middle-aged and overweight men and 350 women achieved, on average, a 4-kilogram (kg) (8.8 lb) weight loss in one year.

They maintained a 3.5-kg (7.7 lb) weight loss during the second year of the study, as well. At the end of the second year, the risk of these individuals' developing diabetes was reduced by 58%!

A second study was conducted in the United States. A large multicenter trial, called the Diabetes Prevention Program, enrolled 3,234 participants with impaired glucose tolerance (IGT), a condition that commonly leads to diabetes. On a low-fat diet, and with exercise of 150 minutes each week, these individuals also reduced their risk of developing diabetes by 58%!

Splendid, wonderful, and encouraging news for Mr. K.! His chances of winning his battle with his early diabetes are greater than 50%!

Diet

Mr. K. weighs 230 pounds and is 6 feet tall. Because his ideal body weight is approximately 180 pounds, he has a long way to go.

If we establish a 50-pound weight reduction as our initial goal, we will most likely fail. This goal is simply unrealistic at this point. We should be much more modest and set our goal at a 20-pound weight loss within the first year, getting Mr. K. down to 210 pounds.

This will be a loss of approximately 8% of his starting weight. If he is successful in attaining this goal and maintaining his reduced weight, we might revise our goals and expectations, but, for now, this 8% weight loss seems to be a realistic and achievable goal.

The very first thing I want Mr. K. to do is to keep a precise list of what he eats—a diary, or "dietary recall," as it is called. Whatever food item makes its way to Mr. K.'s mouth has to be recorded in his food diary. This is the only way to objectively monitor what he eats, to analyze his caloric intake, and to make appropriate adjustments.

After a certain period of time under my guidance, he will learn to make these adjustments on his own. Some people object to keeping such a list, arguing that this exercise focuses them on their problems, instead of allowing them to live free of them. I believe that maintaining this list strengthens our commitment to weight reduction goals. After all, we are on a lifelong mission to change the way we eat and the way we live.

At the same time, I will ask Mr. K. to eliminate from his home, and from his diet, margarine, candies, pastries, flour, sugar, cereals, sour cream, whipped cream, pasta, beer, and all other items that contain more than 6 grams of sugar and/or 2 grams of saturated fat per serving. I also want Mr. K. and his wife to spend an hour, twice a week, in their favorite grocery store, reading and comparing labels of various food items—those that they used to buy and those that they will be buying from now on. They must understand what they are purchasing.

I invited Mrs. K. to accompany her husband to his next appointment with me. She is an integral member of our team, and her support, understanding, and cooperation are absolutely critical. Table 12.1 is a sample menu that the three of us decided would be acceptable for Mr. K.

A number of variations can be introduced to this basic menu, but the goal remains the same—to design a hypocaloric diet containing no more than eighteen Draznin Calories a day (between 1,500 and 1,800 calories) with moderate amounts of carbohydrates.

Table 12.1. Sample Menu for Mr. K.

Breakfast

One soft- or hard-boiled egg (can be pan-fried with a non-stick spray)

One slice of whole wheat bread or toast (preferably low-calorie bread)

½ cup of berries or 2 slices of melon

Water, tea, or coffee

Mid-morning snack

Cup of tea with 1 small apple or with 5 almonds or a slice of cheese

Lunch

Big bowl of salad, with low-fat dressing

Grilled chicken or turkey breast or tuna

Water, tea, or diet soda

Mid-Day Snack

8–10 peeled small carrots

1 apple or pear

Water, diet soda, or tea

Dinner

Large salad with low-fat dressing

Grilled meat, poultry, or fish

Steamed or stir-fried vegetables

1 cup of berries or 2 slices of melon or watermelon

Sugarless fruit popsicle

Water, tea, or coffee

Exercise

Jeffrey K. is a very sedentary man, but he does not have any other health problems aside from his recently diagnosed diabetes and mild hypertension. He is also over thirty-five years of age, and I would like to see a normal exercise stress test before recommending an exercise program to him, even one as simple as three Draznin Miles.

Once the stress test clears him for an exercise program, he can easily start his way to the three Draznin Miles a day program. He can accomplish this by walking ten minutes away from his home and ten minutes back, twice a day. I want him to do this for three weeks, and then increase his walking distance to fifteen minutes each way.

This would translate into an hour a day of walking! This is a great goal for the next couple of months. The magic three Draznin Miles a day are within his reach.

Meanwhile, I want Mr. K. to buy a pair of new and comfortable walking shoes and a pedometer. Realizing that the goal is to take at least 10,000 to 11,000 steps daily, he should know where he stands right now, and the progress he will be making on his way to the goal. I firmly believe that even a small investment will offer a huge boost to his motivation.

Lifestyle

Changing his diet and embarking on a walking program are already great improvements in Mr. K.'s lifestyle. But we want more. Fortunately, he does not smoke, and he drinks only minimal amounts of wine. I do not believe it will be difficult for him to abstain from alcohol. I want Mr. and Mrs. K. to find out what kinds of meditation and yoga classes are available in their community. I want them to visit some of these programs and speak to the instructors. We will discuss their findings about a month from now, when they are somewhat adjusted to their new diet and exercise routine.

We shake hands, and Mr. K. leaves my office. He will return in a week (after his exercise test) with Mrs. K. and an initial report on his progress. He will certainly bring the list of food items he has eaten during the week. We will recheck his blood-sugar level and blood pressure and spend some time together. We will have taken the first 2 steps on his long road to success.

Recommendations Based on Ten Draznin Rules of Life

Science is the orderly arrangement of what, at the moment, seem to be the facts.

(*Anonymous*)

Recommendation 1

Three Draznin miles and fewer than eighteen Draznin calories a day are the keys to your successful fight with obesity and diabetes.

Recommendation 2

Select a knowledgeable doctor who has both the interest and the time to discuss your lifestyle problems with you.

Recommendation 3

Develop a set of reasonable goals, and achieve them one by one.

Recommendation 4

Do not stay on a very low calorie diet for more than ten days. Rather, always be on a hypocaloric diet that has been developed to meet your goals.

Recommendation 5

Always stay on a low-carbohydrate diet, unless your BMI is under 25 and you do at least six Draznin miles a day.

Recommendation 6

Exclude saturated fat from your diet, but do not be afraid of mono- and polyunsaturated fats. Remember that a Mediterranean diet based on these fats is both healthy and tasty.

Recommendation 7

Never eat or drink anything that contains more than 6 grams of sugar per serving.

Recommendation 8

Remember that, at every stage of your life, you are personally responsible for at least 90% of its quality.

Recommendation 9

He who would eat the kernel must crack the nut. You must have a lifelong commitment to your lifestyle choices. It is never too late to start your commitment.

Recommendation 10

Never forget Recommendation 1!

Frequently
Asked
Questions

People in general, and my patients are not an exception, always have questions about their health. I do everything possible to encourage my patients not only to generate these questions, but to bring them to my attention. Their questions reflect the individuality of their problems and, it is hoped, my answers boost their confidence, adherence to, and compliance with their treatment plans. What follows are typical questions my patients ask followed by my short answers that might also be helpful to you. I will also tell you how to contact me and other sources to help answer questions and concerns you have.

Question 1. I started on your program about three months ago and I am still doing fairly well with the dietary part.

However, it's the walking part that gives me trouble. I've built up my walking program to twenty minutes a day, and I just don't seem to have time either in the morning or in the evening to increase my exercise. I leave home early, return about 6, we eat dinner at 6:30 or 7, and after dinner I am too tired to go out. I watch TV for about an hour, and then read in bed for about twenty to thirty minutes. Do you have any suggestions as to how I can deal with my problem?

Answer 1. I understand that you have a long workday and find it difficult to squeeze more exercise into your day. Several ways are available to deal with this. First, there is a wonderful program developed at the University of Colorado Health Science Center under the direction of Dr. James Hill. Participants are asked to wear a pedometer, a little gizmo that is worn on the belt and counts the number of steps one makes. After a week, a staff member calculates the average number of steps the participant did daily and asks him or her to add 2,000 steps every day. These 2,000 steps can be made at any time during the day; They can come from walking an extra flight of stairs, parking your car farther away in the parking lot and walking the extra distance, or making another circle around the park. The 2,000 steps represent about one mile, and adding them to your daily walking regimen can go a long way toward your three Draznin miles a day.

The second way of finding time to exercise is to use the time you watch TV. This way is a bit more expensive. You should purchase a treadmill, place it in front of your TV and use it while watching your favorite program. Personally, if I watch a sporting event, I do it only while walking on my treadmill.

Question 2. I have noticed that lately both my husband and I feel extremely anxious about several things in our lives: things like job security, pension funds, our teenage children, and our elderly parents. Every time I worry about one of these things, I feel hungry, I eat, and, not surprisingly, I have gained weight. Is there a relationship between anxiety and weight gain?

Answer 2. Very much so, even though no one knows the exact nature of this relationship. Conceivably, chemical and/or hormonal imbalance in the brain can be the culprit. Brain cells misfire, disconnect, lose inhibitory control, and become incompetent in regulating the sense of satiety. At the same time, anxiety can be accompanied by increased output of adrenalin, which can change the levels of glucose in the blood and consequently the levels of insulin and the sensation of hunger.

Let me share with you a story about my patient, Mr. Zi. Mr. Zi is a private investigator who also repossesses automobiles on behalf of lenders when people default on their loans. He converted a process of repossession into an art of towing away a car within forty-five seconds, a sort of legalized car theft. During these quick operations (they must be quick to avoid an altercation with an irate owner), he is focused, concentrated on his task, and extremely anxious. Approximately twenty to thirty minutes after the towing, he feels thirsty and extremely hungry. Mr. Zi has gained over 30 pounds in the span of two years, despite being reasonably active at work and in the gym.

I believe the treatment of anxiety and elimination of anxiety-provoking factors should come first, before any successful diet can be instituted.

Question 3. Every day I try to eat a light lunch, such as a salad or just a cup of soup. I feel fine for about an hour or two, but then I become terribly hungry. I can no longer concentrate on my work. I go through our large office searching for candies or cookies that many of my co-workers keep around. I tried bringing some fruit from home, but this didn't help, I was still extremely hungry. How shall I deal with my bouts of mid-afternoon hunger?

Answer 3. This is probably the biggest problem with dieting. Regardless of the type of diet we follow, when we become hungry it is very difficult to adhere to any program. Hunger is a dominant feeling. When we are really hungry, our mind is completely preoccupied with food. The thought of subsequent regret is driven away; the hunger prevails, and behavior is dominated by a search for food. We become overwhelmed by the hunger-driven inability to maintain our dietary program.

I must say at the outset, this problem is extremely common and there is nothing to be ashamed of. It is also a losing proposition trying to fight one's hunger by evoking the remnants of one's willpower. The only way to succeed is to change the environment in which we find ourselves at the time we feel hungry, to get away from food and to switch our mind to something completely different that can occupy us for a while.

I recommend the minute you feel this uncontrollable hunger (after that small lunch that you were supposed to eat to stay on your diet) to leave your house, if you are at home. Go for a walk, go to the library, a bookstore, a department store, a museum—anywhere to be away from food and, better yet, where your mind can become engaged in a totally new activity, such as reading, analyzing, comparing, calculating, making plans, and so forth.

Certainly, this is much harder to do at work. When you remain hungry after lunch, sitting at your desk with your mind overwhelmed with thoughts of food, first try sipping water or a noncaloric drink. Frequently, small sips curb your feeling of hunger. If this doesn't help, a dozen almonds or a stick of string cheese is the next line of defense. Still the best approach to this residual hunger is to get truly busy and to be away from food. Schedule a meeting, discuss work-related problems, get busy with manual tasks, do anything that takes your mind away from food.

Question 4. Someone told me that eating twice a day is the best way to lose weight. I tried this but found it difficult not to eat between breakfast and dinner. What is a good interval of time between meals?

Answer 4. I recommend that you eat every five to six hours during daytime. For example, eat at 8 A.M., 1 P.M., and 6 to 7 P.M. I also stress that the time interval between the end of your dinner and your next breakfast be no less than twelve hours. If you finish your dinner at 8 P.M., do not eat your breakfast before 8 A.M. the next morning.

Question 5. I've been looking for a diet that I can stick to without making a huge effort to find the "right" food items or perfect cooking style. What is the simplest and the most effective diet for a man who wants to lose 10 to 15 pounds?

Answer 5. The Draznin Calorie plan allows you to eat any grilled low-fat meat, poultry, or fish with most of the vegetables (except potatoes and corn) and a variety of fruit (except grapes and bananas). If you stay with these recommendations, you will lose 10 to 15 pounds within 3 months easily.

Question 6. I weigh 265 pounds and I have Type 2 diabetes that I am treating with a total of 114 units of insulin taken in three separate injections. I am ready to go on a strict low-calorie diet. How do I adjust my insulin? Do I stop it altogether?

Answer 6. Most likely you can cut your insulin dose in half without any problems, provided you are serious about trimming your food intake and that you measure your blood sugar levels four times a day. Several years ago my colleagues and I conducted a study in which we recommended our overweight diabetic patients to be on a five-day fast, drinking only noncaloric fluids, before initiating dietary therapy. These patients did not take any insulin during this complete five-day fast, and they resumed taking it afterwards depending upon their blood-sugar readings. These patients did very well, and only half of them required insulin after this initial fast. The danger arises if you reduce your insulin dose but do not reduce what you eat and do not check your blood-sugar levels. Clearly, working with your doctor or diabetes educator is preferable to doing it alone.

Question 7. I am 5 foot 6 and weigh 208 pounds. I am taking two pills for my lipids, two for diabetes, two for high blood pressure, one aspirin, and multivitamins. I have recently gained 7 pounds and my blood sugar is just above 200 mg/dl. I was told to start taking another medication that might prevent absorption of sugars. Is there another way to achieve better control of my problems without so many pills?

Answer 7. Losing weight will help tremendously. Most likely your diabetes will improve and quite likely your blood pressure and lipids will also improve. You seem to be a prime candidate for the Draznin Plan if you are ready to embark on this program. I also recommend meditation classes for mild hypertension and for learning to take control of your problems.

Question 8. I work out in the gym three times a week and I cut down on the carbohydrates in my diet. I am really trying to eat healthy—fruits and vegetables. I drink a lot of fruit juices, not sodas, four to six glasses of orange or cranberry juice a day. Yet I have lost only 2 pounds in the last four months. Is there anything else I should be doing?

Answer 8. Unfortunately, yours is a common mistake. Fruit juices are extremely caloric, with simple sugars accounting for most of the calories. I firmly recommend that any fluid you consume (except for milk) should contain *no* calories. Stopping fruit juices would be my immediate recommendation.

Question 9. I followed your program for over six months and I lost 18 pounds. I now weigh 192 pounds, down from 210. I walk an hour every day, but during the last three weeks I haven't lost any more weight. How do I get on the weight-losing track again?

Answer 9. An excellent question. Remember, the first goal of the Draznin Plan is to help you lose about 10% of your initial weight and maintain the reduced weight for about six to twelve months. At this point, one must re-evaluate the program and make the next step. For example, if you are not doing three Draznin Miles a day, you should make an effort to get to this goal. If you do, you might want to increase your walking or jogging speed or possibly extend the time by an additional ten minutes a day. You can add 2,000 steps daily or be a little stricter about your diet.

Question 10. I have learned to take boredom out of my daily walks—I listen to books on tape as I stroll through our neighborhood, around a small park, and back home. It works well. It's the dietary part that I find more difficult to follow, simply because my choices are somewhat limited. In other words, the diet is boring. What would you suggest?

Answer 10. I would recommend expanding the variety of meat or fish you are buying and of the vegetables you eat. There are wonderful recipes in vegetarian cookbooks that you can adopt as well as numerous types of fish and nonfat meat that you can grill or sear. Adding various spices may also help.

Question 11. My blood sugar levels hover around 220 mg/dl. My doctor tried me on three different medications, but they didn't seem to help. My weight is 190 pounds, and my doctor tells me that unless I lose weight, he will have to start me on insulin. Is there anything else I can do?

Answer 11. Your doctor is absolutely correct to suggest that controlling your blood sugar is your number-one priority. However, you can help yourself and your doctor to accomplish this task by losing weight. In this case, you may avoid insulin altogether. A lot of it is in your own hands.

Question 12. My twenty-two-year-old daughter weighs 186 pounds and is only 5 feet 4 inches tall. Most importantly, however, she refuses to do anything about her weight. She says she feels good about herself, enjoys her friends and her lifestyle, and is proud to be who she is. On the one hand, I am glad she is not depressed and that she maintains her self-confidence; on the other hand, I am very much concerned and don't know how to help her. Your advice?

Answer 12. Unfortunately, your ability to help is limited at this point. A direct discussion or repeated confrontations will not help. You might work indirectly, so to speak. Invite her for walks, hikes, bike rides, or a swim. Change the way you cook at home, and, it is hoped, she will like the new recipes. Suggest that she consult a psychologist, perhaps for some other reason (if such exists), and then recommend to your daughter that she talk with the psychologist about her weight. This is not an easy task; it will certainly take some time, but being concerned about it is the first step.

Question 13. If I have a question about my weight maintenance or my diabetes, how can I contact you?

Answer 13. You can find me at the University of Colorado Health Sciences Center. In addition, you can obtain valuable information from numerous excellent Web sites related to diabetes, appropriately led by the American Diabetes Association (www.diabetes.org), Juvenile Diabetes Federation (www. jdf.org); International Diabetes Federation (www.idf.org); British Diabetes Association (www.diabetes.org.uk); and the Joslin Diabetes Center (www.joslin.harvard.edu).

Index